This book is

- You had a lockdown baby
- You didn't have a lockdown baby so can laugh and breathe a sigh of relief
- You want the truth about the first year
- You like a giggle
- You sometimes feel like you're doing too many things and none of them well
- You lost yourself in motherhood but also found yourself
- You need to know we're all in it together
- You're basically just winging it!

What people are saying....

"A tell-it-how-it-is mum must read. An acutely honest, sharp, witty, and perceptive dive into the realities of modern motherhood. A light-hearted and comforting reminder that we're all in this together."

"A joyous account of becoming a mum of four that every parent will be able to relate to. It's full of laughter and love but doesn't shy away from telling the sometimes brutal truth about pregnancy, childbirth and parenting."

"From the madness of the Tupperware perfect weaning we think is required to be a good mummy to the horrors that were homeschooling, there's something everyone can relate to whether you have one child or six."

Unashamedly oversharing the truth about the first year.

Confessions of a Crummy Mummy - The Baby Years by parenting blogger and accidental mum of four Natalie Brown (@ confessionsofacrummymummy) is the literary equivalent of the tea and toast you're handed after giving birth: warm, reassuring and you can't help but want more!

An antidote to the traditional parenting manual, the telling-it-how-it-is parenting memoir lifts the lid on a subject the hugely successful genre of telling-it-how-it-is parenting memoirs has yet to touch on: giving birth during a global pandemic. And let's just say giving birth during a global pandemic was *not* in the birth plan!

An easy-to-digest and quick-paced list-style format offers a collection of witty and brutally honest confessions time-poor mums can dip in and out of and back into again.

About the Author

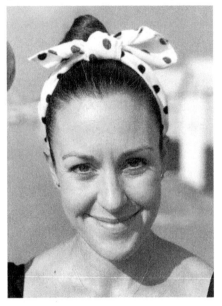

Natalie Brown is a wife, mother, freelance journalist, and blogger – not necessarily in that order! She started blogging under the pseudonym Confessions of a Crummy Mummy in 2013 while on maternity leave from her job as a local newspaper editor and finding herself with lots to say and nobody to say it to.

Three more babies, more nappies than she can possibly count, and *lots* of wine later she is now an accidental mum of four who has been there, done it and got the (sick stained) t-shirt, most recently during lockdown when her fourth and final maternity leave was hijacked by three kids, a husband on a short fuse, homeschooling, and trying to find the right Zoom codes. And yes that *is* as scary as it sounds!

You can follow her everyday parenting adventures on Instagram and Facebook

@confessionsofacrummymummy
and Twitter
@mrsnataliebrown

www.crummymummy.co.uk

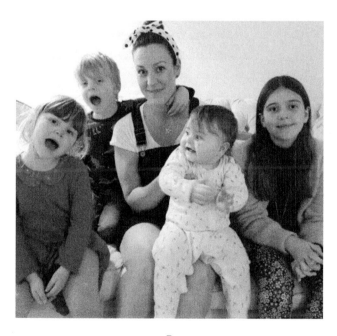

Dedication

For Bluebell, Maximilian,
Marigold, and Violet,
without whom this book
wouldn't have been possible

(And for Misery Guts,
who *may* have had a
small part to play)

Confessions of a CRUMMY MUMMY

The Baby Years

Unashamedly oversharing the truth about the first year

Natalie Brown

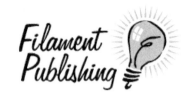

Published by
Filament Publishing Ltd
16, Croydon Road, Beddington,
Croydon, Surrey CR0 4PA   UK
www.filamentpublishing.com
+44 (0)20 6882498

ISBN 978-1-913623-60-9

Confessions of a Crummy Mummy - The Baby Years
by Natalie Brown

Contents

"Let's just say giving birth in a global pandemic was not in the birth plan!"

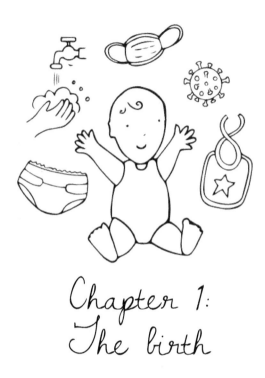

Chapter 1:
The birth

Confessions from the head end: a hospital on divert, a flashing fuel light, and giving birth in a global pandemic.

If you'd told me after the birth of my first child that I'd one day be a mother of four I'd have laughed so hard tears would have run down my legs. At 10.58 am on Monday, August 15th, 2011 - one minute after my first daughter Bluebell Rose was born following a wildly painful induction - I vowed I'd never, ever do *that* again.

By *that* I mean pushing a human being out of my lady bits. Which despite a small fortune spent on antenatal classes coupled with the first-hand experience of equally unwitting mamas I met at those classes *nothing* fully prepares you for.

Because it turns out there's an awful lot they don't tell you about giving birth, things that afterwards I felt quite frankly outraged nobody was honest enough to warn me about. Like floating turds, bags of wee and green placentas.

The thing is I did do it again - in 2014, 2017, and (accidentally) in 2020, at the height of the first wave of the coronavirus pandemic. And let's just say giving birth in a global pandemic was *not* in the birth plan!

I finished work to go on maternity leave the day schools and nurseries across the UK closed for what we now know was Lockdown 1, and I finished maternity leave to go back to work nine months later on the day schools closed for Lockdown 3. Owing to the various lockdowns and tiers in between all in all I had just three months of my nine months maternity leave on my own with our lockdown baby Violet Hope. The rest is a blur of home learning grids, trying to find the right Zoom code and Joe Wicks, who, owing to the fact we live in a fourth-floor flat with noise-sensitive neighbours, I could have cheerfully throttled. It's fair to say I'm the sort of person who always gets pooed on (I don't just mean by little people, I mean by birds – it *always* happens to me) and when it came to my last maternity leave it's fair to say I was well and truly shat on from a great height.

So, after four babies - including an accidental lockdown one - here's what I wish I'd known about the birth:

1. Expect the unexpected.

Like babies that don't want to be born, babies that *do* want to be born, a hospital on divert and a husband who forgets to fill the car with fuel. Oh, and the small matter of a global pandemic. Luckily not all at the same time.

To be honest, the phrase expect the unexpected can be applied to the whole of motherhood, but it turns out it starts well before they're actually born. For me that was 15 days after my due date with Bluebell, who didn't want to budge despite all the old wives' tales: bouncing around like a maniac on a birthing ball; rogan josh; pineapple juice; a bit of how's your father; then - in desperation - bouncing around like a maniac on a birthing ball *with* a rogan josh *and* pineapple juice *and* a bit of how's your father. None of which worked.

Induction was the only thing for it – and my intricate and detailed plan for a natural water birth disappeared down the plug hole along with the birthing pool water I never used. But more on all that later - let's just say the baby I *thought* would glide naturally into the world to the dulcet tones of a carefully choreographed playlist didn't, and needed rather a lot more persuading.

Ironically, the exact opposite happened when it came to her brother Max, our rainbow baby after two consecutive miscarriages, three years later. He couldn't *wait* to be born – which I wasn't expecting at all. But it was baby number three Marigold, two years after that on Valentine's Day 2017 (she'll probably hate us for that one day) when things really got interesting. You'd *think* having been there, done it and got the sick-stained t-shirt twice before that we'd be prepared for anything, but nope.

After days of stop-start labour, I was so convinced the whole process would be as long and drawn out as it was the first time around that I waited until the last possible minute to call the hospital five minutes up the road to say it might be a good idea to come in now. Only to discover there was no room at the inn and the labour ward was on divert – to a hospital in a different county 40 minutes away. And there's a *big* difference between a hospital in a different county 40 minutes away and one five minutes up the road when you've got a baby intent on making an appearance.

Unsurprisingly this sent Misery Guts (I'll introduce you to him properly later) into a spin, flinging towels out of the airing cupboard for the journey 'just in case'. And he was right to fly into a panic. What he knew but I was yet to find out is that the fuel warning light was flashing on the car - and had been for quite some time. And there was no way it was going to get us to the hospital 40 minutes away without going via a garage first.

Now, any mama will tell you that being strapped into a car while in labour is the *last* place you want to be, and the sooner you can get from A to B the better. But take it from me: the unforgiving lights of a garage forecourt while a hapless teenager looks on from the night hatch is worse, *especially* if you're about to push a human being out of your own night hatch.

I'd also recommend knowing how to get to the hospital 40 minutes away because googling the route while actually *en route* and in labour is a very bad idea. We did eventually make it to the hospital in time, but that flashing fuel light still bugs me, in the same infuriating way as recreating an argument you had years ago but with new and better points.

I had spent nine months growing a human being, enduring the all-day hell of 'morning' sickness – not to mention eye watering acid reflux and night sweats – all while going without the niceties of life like pate, mould-ripened cheese, and – more importantly – wine. I hadn't slept properly for months, couldn't see my lady bits and had to grunt when sitting down and getting up. And now I was faced with the prospect of pushing that human being out of my foo-foo – possibly in the back of a car with the help of someone who couldn't even be relied on to fill a car with fuel. All *he* had to do was make sure the car was filled with enough diesel to get us to the hospital. It's not too much to ask, is it?

On the upside, while flinging towels out of the airing cupboard he also had the foresight to fling my Valentine's Day card and present *into* the hospital bag, because by then it was clear that we were going to have a Valentine's Day baby. And when he produced them shortly after the birth in the early hours of Valentine's Day I forgot all about the flashing fuel light. Temporarily.

But flashing fuel lights pale into insignificance compared to what happened next: accidentally giving birth in a global pandemic. When I first saw the thin blue line appear on my pregnancy test in August 2019 not only did the prospect of having four kids seem ludicrous (because three is the magic number and I hadn't heard the saying one's lonely, two fight, three's piggy in the middle, four's just right yet). I could never have *dreamed* of the world my baby would be born into just eight months later. The concept of lockdown alone sounded like a plot for a film.

But a lot can happen in nine months - and I don't just mean growing a human being. With a full-scale national lockdown on the horizon, I finished work to go on maternity leave the day schools and nurseries across the UK closed, and I watched my fourth and final maternity leave go down the plug hole, a bit like the birthing pool water I never got to use the first time around.

The highly anticipated naps, daytime TV and tea and cake in coffee shops while the kids were at school and nursery and I rested and waited for my baby to arrive were replaced with home learning grids, daily government briefings, and banana bread that I had to not only referee the baking of but the clearing up of the bombsite formerly known as the kitchen afterwards. Not to mention the four breakfasts, lunches with starters, main courses and desserts and two million snacks I was suddenly expected to produce every day. Who knew kids could eat so much? They say free school meals save a family £400 a year but is that *all*? At one point we were on our third loaf of bread by a Wednesday.

It was about then that I realised living in a two-bedroom flat with no garden and three kids, two cats, a newborn baby and a husband on a short fuse trying to work in one of the bedrooms was either going to make or break us. The one permitted trip outside a day during Lockdown 1 became a lifeline, and suddenly the prospect of having baby number four was the least of my worries. I thought accidentally having a fourth baby was going to be the biggest thing to happen to us in 2020, but it turns out Covid was. And I think we can all agree there was nothing more unexpected than that.

2. Giving birth in a global pandemic isn't as scary as it sounds.

Even though the whole country was in lockdown, even though maternity unit guidelines were changing by the hour and even though I went from being able to visualise everything about the birth to not being able to picture it at all, giving birth in lockdown isn't as scary as it sounds.

The truth is the run-up to the birth and the anxiety

about what may or may not happen was worse than actually giving birth in a pandemic, because the one constant you're fed from the moment you discover you're pregnant is that it's your body, your baby, your choice. Except suddenly it wasn't, and many of the choices we previously took for granted like birth partners and labour options were snatched away, and no one could really say for sure what would and wouldn't be allowed on the big day.

Could Misery Guts be there? Would I have to labour alone? Worse, would I actually have to give birth alone? What would happen if a member of our household displayed coronavirus symptoms? Would I still be able to have a water birth? Would I have to wear PPE gear? Who was going to look after the kids when I went into labour? Would my mum and dad get stopped by the police if they came to help? How was I going to manage home schooling two while entertaining a three-year-old and looking after a newborn? Would I ever sleep again?

These were the questions going through my mind and keeping me awake in the small hours in the run-up to the birth, and I cried more in the last month of my pregnancy than I have in the last 10 years. I could have cheerfully throttled people who said things like 'what a terrible time to be giving birth' and 'if I were you, I wouldn't go *near* a hospital right now,' as if I'd planned it.

By the time I did finally go into labour, at the height of the first wave of the pandemic on Monday, April 20th, 2020, it was actually a relief because it meant the worrying – and the unhelpful unsolicited advice – would finally come to an end.

As it was the whole thing was (rather disappointingly) uneventful. There was no hospital on divert or flashing fuel lights, no grandparents getting stopped by police for crossing county borders and no husband forced to wait outside in a hospital car park. My parents made it from their house to our house in record time owing to lockdown and the fact there were fewer cars on the road, and Misery Guts was allowed to be with me for the birth and for a few hours afterwards just like he had been with the other three. The only real difference, other than midwives in full PPE gear, was that I was only allowed to labour in water but not give birth in the pool owing to continually changing health and safety guidelines. So, not as scary as it sounds.

The scary bit came when we arrived home from the hospital and it dawned on me I had four kids including a newborn baby to look after, my maternity leave had not only been hijacked but completely ruined, home schooling two while entertaining a three-year-old and looking after a newborn was going to be impossible because that's a job for at least three people and as far as sleeping goes, forget it.

The low point – and there were *lots* of low points - is the day all six of us were crying. All at the same time. I can't remember about what specifically – I've blocked that bit out – but I was done mumming, Misery Guts was done dadding, the kids were done kidding and the baby was done babying. Basically, we had all had enough todaying that day. And that *is* as scary as it sounds.

3. Birth plans don't tend to go to plan.

In fact, I don't think I know anyone whose birth plan has gone to plan. Because there are certain things you just can't plan for, like the aforementioned babies that don't want to be born, babies that *do* want to be born, hospitals on divert and global pandemics. (You can, of course, plan for flashing fuel lights. Just saying).

I can't tell you how much time I spent on my birth plan with baby number one. I even wrote out several versions on separate bits of paper first so it would be perfect by the time I transferred The One to my maternity notes. I was *that* mama who not only filled the entire page and wrote in the margin with asterisks but attached extra sheets to cover various different scenarios. None of which ever became a reality.

Going into labour naturally, labouring at home for as long as possible, and transferring to the hospital and the tranquillity of a birthing pool for a drug-free labour turned into cannulas, catheters, epidurals, heart monitors, and more tubes than you can shake a stick at.

So I didn't bother with baby number two – which is just as well because he came so quickly my maternity notes were still waiting patiently on a desk somewhere in the depths of triage and the midwife had to write all his vital signs down on a napkin. And I didn't bother with baby number three, or baby number four. And that was just as well too given we were in the middle of a pandemic and nobody could plan anything then, not even the midwives. The situation was changing faster than Boris's daily briefings.

4. It hurts. *A lot.*

And nobody tells you how much. Not your midwife, not the internet, not your mum and not your mum friends. Because the fact is words simply *cannot* describe just how painful labour is.

And even if they can, no one wants to be the one to tell you.

I wondered after the birth of baby number one whether I'd simply been naïve in not appreciating *quite* how much it was going to hurt. Or hadn't been listening properly in the antenatal classes when they talked about rings of fire. But it wasn't either of those things.

After four babies – one of whom was born with the help of an epidural and three of whom I somehow managed to produce completely drug-free – I can confirm it hurts *waay* more than you think it's going to. Think about how much you *think* it's going to hurt, times that by ten, then times that number by ten and you'll be somewhere closer to the truth.

The truth is giving birth is the hardest day's work you'll ever do in your entire life. Or several days if you're especially unlucky. *Nothing* compares. You'll find strength and resilience you never knew existed, never mind that you possessed, and it's only when you're in the throes of it all that you truly understand the concept of animal instinct. Because there's *nothing* on this earth as fierce and mighty as a mama about to give birth.

5. Epidurals are The. Best. Thing. Ever.

I was heavily pregnant with baby number one when someone advised me not to 'martyr myself' and accept all the pain relief that was on offer. I vividly recall inwardly turning my nose up at the prospect of an epidural, because epidurals are a cop-out and for wimps, right? *Wrong!* They might have a stigma attached but epidurals are not a cop-out and they're not for wimps, either. Epidurals are one of the best things ever invented, taking the pain they don't tell you about from ten to nought in a matter of minutes.

It was only when I surprised myself by going into labour naturally and having Max completely drug-free without any form of pain relief that I realised just how much epidurals get an unfairly bad press. The pain I experienced as a result of being induced with Bluebell was so far removed from the pain I experienced – and breathed through without any drugs at all – with Max that it's almost impossible to put into words.

Induction is a bit like a switch being flicked and going from nought to ten in the pain stakes, and afterwards I was left with an overwhelming sense of failure at having 'resorted to' an epidural. Because having an epidural isn't technically classed as a natural birth. It's a 'medically assisted' one.

Yet there's absolutely nothing natural about being induced, and if there's nothing natural about being induced, then why on earth would you endure it 'naturally'?

It was only after three 'natural' births that I realised I hadn't failed in my 'medically assisted' one at all. I simply couldn't have delivered baby number one without the help of an epidural. And there's no badge for no pain relief. So my advice - as I was so sagely advised - is this: don't martyr yourself.

6. You'll poo without even realising it.

It's the last taboo, the horror to end all horrors and the thing I spent my entire first pregnancy worrying about: pooing in front of my other half. Forget birth plans and hospitals on divert and flashing fuel lights and global pandemics: in the run-up to the birth the prospect of pooing in front of Misery Guts and midwives armed with fishing nets haunted me on an almost daily basis. The shame! And the indignity!

What I didn't realise at the time, though, is that I needn't have wasted the time worrying about it. Because when it comes to having a baby you leave your dignity at the door, along with all the preconceived ideas you had about childbirth. And when it actually comes down to it, pooing in front of your other half is the *least* of your worries.

The fact is you won't even know you've done it until it's too late and there it is, floating nonchalantly at eye level in the birthing pool next to you. You'll even wonder who it belongs to and how on earth it got there. And then the realisation dawns on you, but the funny thing is by then you don't care because all you want is for the baby to exit the building, and anything that helps make that happen, like a good clear out, is a good thing.

Until you find yourself unwittingly giving birth in the middle of a global pandemic, that is. Then pooing in the birthing pool is a very *bad* thing because it means you'll have to get out of the pool and have the baby on dry land owing to indeterminate new health and safety guidelines no one really understands. Ironically, in the end, it was Violet who pooed during labour, not me, so I had to get out of the water anyway - which takes us back to my very first point: expect the unexpected.

7. There are things you'll never unsee – and nor will they.

Like the aforementioned floating turds, bags of wee and green placentas. Before giving birth for the first time I thought catheters were something only old people had when they start having problems downstairs. I had *no idea* that having an epidural meant I had to be catheterised too, and that I'd spend the rest of the labour with a bag of my own wee hanging down the side of the bed. Of course, it makes perfect sense when you think about it – the whole point of an epidural is so you don't feel anything from the waist down, bladder included – but the trouble is I *didn't* think about it. And nor did he. There was no dog-eared antenatal class card for that one. The fact is you'll never unsee those bags of wee silently and mysteriously filling up all by themselves, or the nurse who comes along, whips them away and replaces them with an empty one.

And you can never unsee the placenta, which midwives seem to take an almost perverse interest in examining. If you haven't had the pleasure yet delivering the placenta is a bit like giving birth to another baby. Based on size and weight alone it essentially *is* another baby - one they didn't warn you about. And the feeling afterwards, when you've pushed it out, is *amazing*.

It's then the midwife's job to check it's all intact, which in my experience involves holding it up to the light or window and dangling it in front of you to give it the once over. I'll never forget the look of horror on Misery Guts' face. To be fair a placenta isn't something you want to spend too much time looking at, but take it from me, a green one *definitely* isn't.

When baby number four arrived, the midwife got quite excited when instead of the usual burnt umber my placenta was green. She proceeded to go to great lengths to point out the curious hue to everyone who came into the room, and it turns out that because Violet had pooed on her way out the placenta had done exactly what it was supposed to do and filtered all the nasties out – turning it green in the process.

But floating turds, bags of wee and green placentas are nothing when it comes to the first time you stand up after giving birth. Why don't they warn you about that? Baby number three was particularly memorable when the birthing suite looked like someone had been murdered. It was like a scene from a horror film, with blood splattered up the sides of the birthing pool and trailing across the floor from the pool to the bed. There's so much blood you'd think you'd either pass out or die.

What's equally shocking is that no one else bats an eyelid, apart from your other half or whoever has the misfortune to be with you for the birth. They, like you, can never unsee that much blood either. And not only do the midwives not bat an eyelid, the speed and efficiency with which they clear it all up, as though nothing had ever happened, is nothing short of a miracle.

A bit like the placenta examining after baby number four, my midwife after baby number three took an almost perverse pleasure in mopping up the mess, cheerfully telling me what she was going to have for dinner while squeezing my blood from a mop head in a bucket of red water.

8. In the first 10 minutes after the birth you can call the baby whatever you want.

Which is super helpful if you can't agree on a name. And super helpful if they start suggesting corona related ones like Covid and Rona. Luckily, while you're still reeling from the enormity of what just happened, so's he – and he's so in awe of what you've just done that what you say goes. (This is also a jolly good time to get your way on anything else you can't agree on too).

We ended up with:

- a Bluebell Rose (he chose the first name after his favourite flower and was adamant about it from the moment we found out we were expecting. I thought it sounded ridiculous, like the sort of thing the Beckham's might choose, and loved Isabella, but was put off when there were at least five different Isabella's in the school Christmas nativity play picture spread we did in the local newspaper I edited at the time. So I kept coming back to Bluebell too, and I chose her second name after my favourite flower. And yes the combination *did* go down like a lead balloon in some quarters)
- a Maximilian James (I chose the first name after Bavarian kings because I love Bavaria – in fact, it's where Misery Guts proposed – and because it sounds strong and I like the letter x. Which sounds ridiculous I know, but the letter x does have a certain ring to it. James is a family name – it's one of Misery Guts' middle names and also my brother's name)
- a Marigold May (think Lady Edith's illegitimate daughter Miss Marigold in Downton Abbey; May because we liked the alliteration. We call her Maggie May after Rod Stewart's song of the same name for short, and the nickname has stuck)
- a Violet Hope (Violet because it's one of the first flowers of spring and with two flower names already we kind of needed to stick with a flower theme; Hope in a nod to the unprecedented time at which she entered the world).

So, if you haven't agreed on names before the big day don't panic – there'll be at least a 10-minute window to get your way. And for those of us who gave birth during the pandemic, a lockdown silver lining was having a bit longer to decide if you couldn't agree on a name because you couldn't register the birth anyway. Usually, births in England, Wales, and Northern Ireland must be registered within 42 days, but during the pandemic, birth registration was suspended, presumably because they were registering so many deaths (it's probably best not to dwell on the whys and why nots). It was 10 weeks – or 70 days – before we were finally able to make Violet official. And as it was we did go for a corona-related name: Violet Hope just seemed right under the circumstances.

9. The best tea and toast you'll ever eat is the tea and toast they give you after giving birth.

Even if the toast is lukewarm and the tea is cold (I think they do it on purpose, just to get you used to every meal you won't eat hot for the next 18 years). In fact, I'd go as far as to say it's the finest meal you will ever eat in your life.

You can smell burnt toast wafting about the labour ward, a silent signal that a baby has just been born, and once you're In The Know the thought – and smell - of that toast is what will get you through those final stages of labour. Then you'll annoy everyone you know by talking about it for the rest of your life.

I'll never forget the tea and toast I was given after each labour and birth. Even the heel I was allocated after the birth of baby number two (under any other circumstances heel toast would be a *big* no-no). And even pandemic toast. In fact, the pandemic toast was the best one, because the harder the labour and birth, the more satisfying the tea and toast.

10. You'll forget all about it.

Not the tea or toast or the momentous bits, like the moment you first set eyes on them or the smell of them. I mean the horrifying bits, like floating turds, bags of wee and green placentas. You'll even forget the fact you did it in the middle of a global pandemic. (Although you won't forget a flashing fuel light).

Because the brain is a clever, funny thing, quite quickly lulling you into a false sense of security that actually, on reflection, *that* wasn't that bad after all. Until you do it all over again and remember that actually it was – and you vow never ever to do that again. Again.

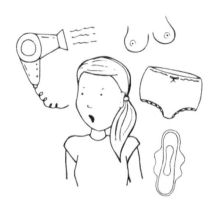

Chapter 2:

Lady bits

Confessions from upstairs and downstairs: queefing, alternative uses for a hair dryer, and embracing the 'new normal'.

Upstairs and downstairs; bits and pieces; carpet and drapes - whatever you call them in your house, I'm talking about lady bits of course. And more specifically what happens to those lady bits when you've grown a human being - or two or three or four - and then pushed them out of your foo-foo.

"You're left to find out for yourself that fanny farting is an occupational hazard of pushing a baby out"

What to expect may be *vaguely* alluded to at antenatal classes and in witty memes on social media, but both often pose more questions than they answer. The truth is no one *really* gives you the lowdown on what to expect in the lady bits department after giving birth, or what to do about it when you're bleeding and aching and stinging and leaking.

You're left to find out for yourself that fanny farting is an occupational hazard of pushing a baby out, and that the best way to dry your foo-foo afterwards is with a hairdryer. The truth is learning to live with the 'new normal' has been a reality for us mamas way before the phrase was coined to describe the aftermath of a global pandemic.

So, after four babies - including an accidental lockdown one - here's what I wish I'd known about my lady bits:

1. Stitches itch. A lot.

And being padded up to the nines with super-size sanitary towels after the birth only makes it worse. Even if you put them in the freezer first (the sanitary towels I mean, not your stitches). Having never had stitches where the sun doesn't shine - or anywhere else - before it was only when trapped in stirrups with legs akimbo that I realised there's also an *awful* lot they don't tell you about stitches downstairs.

Firstly, I had the misfortune of a midwife wearing glasses on two of the three occasions a needle and thread was required to repair the damage. And the trouble with glasses is that you can see everything that's going on in the needlework department reflected in the lenses. And I mean *everything*.

Secondly, if you think pooing in front of your other half is the worst thing that can happen during childbirth, it isn't. Being strapped in stirrups with a spotlight shining on your foof while a team of strangers sews it up is.

I'll never forget the look on Misery Guts' face when he realised this was about to happen right in front of his very eyes, and there was absolutely nowhere he could run to because it was his job to hold the baby. Like me, he just had to grin and bear it. He always wore a hoodie for labour and birth after that, the hood of which he promptly retreated into straight after the delivery with the drawstring cord pulled tight around his face like Kenny from South Park. (If you don't know who Kenny from South Park is ask the internet and you'll see what I mean). And I can't say I blame him, because who in their right mind wants to see a foof being sewn up?

2. A tear is better than a graze.

You'd *think* your foof ripping apart as your bundle of joy enters the world would be worse than a graze, which sounds like something minor that might sting for a bit before you forget all about it. You'd *think*. But the thing is stitches are better than no stitches because then the aforementioned foof starts to heal straight away instead of being left to its own devices.

Having had stitches after baby number one, baby number two, and baby number three (lucky me) it was only after baby number four, when the midwife proudly proclaimed that I had suffered only a 'slight graze', that I discovered a graze is, in fact, *far* worse than a tear. And there's no such thing as a 'slight' graze, either.

What my midwife failed to tell me is that a 'graze' would sting like a b*tch every time I went for a wee, and weeing in my own bath or shower would suddenly become not only perfectly acceptable but the preferred way of doing it.

She failed to tell me I would wince when sitting down and getting up again, and that I would yelp without warning at inopportune moments throughout the day if it happened to twang in the wrong direction.

Which is most unfortunate if you happen to be in a supermarket queue, and downright weird if a lady in that queue gives you a knowing look.

She also failed to tell me you can get spritz especially for your bits, which not only makes you sigh in the same way that first post-pregnancy sip of wine does, but will spray upside down in the downstairs department so it reaches the cupboard *under* the stairs too if you know what I mean. The no man's land that you daren't look at but are quite certain will never be the same again.

I've still got an empty bottle of that spritz for bits in my bedside table drawer. It's next to an empty tube of stretch mark cream, and an empty tub of tummy rub butter. Every now and then I take the lid off the bottle, flip the cap off the tube and unscrew the top of the butter and have a little sniff. Just to remind me of days I had a baby in my tummy and a newborn in my arms. But I digress.

The cynic in me wonders whether the decision not to stitch my 'slight' pandemic graze was a Covid related one, the idea being the less contact with potentially infected mamas and their foofs the better. But I guess we'll never know. Or perhaps we will if it ever transpires there was an unusually high number of mamas twanging in Tesco.

3. Varicose veins don't just happen on legs.

It turns out they can happen on foo-foos too. And mine was purple. I kid you not, this thing with a life of its own appeared out of nowhere shortly after I discovered I was expecting Marigold. It started life as a little niggling caterpillar you wouldn't really know was there but ended up like Julia Donaldson and Axel Scheffler's Superworm - super long and super strong (if you know, you know – if you don't, again, ask the internet and you'll see what I mean). And the bigger the baby got, the bigger superworm got. To the point it practically had its own heartbeat.

After a few sleepless nights worrying about it (because I didn't know what 'it' actually was yet), and after weighing up the pros and cons of consulting Misery Guts but thinking better of it (because as we've already established in confessions from the head end, there are some things you just *can't* unsee) I did The Thing you should never do. I looked it up on the internet. Which, funnily enough, isn't for the faint-hearted.

As well as a collection of increasingly alarming images confirming what I already suspected, that a superworm on your foo-foo is indeed the sort of thing you'll never unsee - *especially* when it's on someone else - it turns out a varicose vein on your foo-foo isn't as weird as it sounds. Except they're not actually called varicose veins at all, even though that's what they are. They're called vulva varicosities. And I don't know about you, but when it comes to lady bits a vulva varicositie has to be The Best Name Ever. The sort of name that makes you want to say it again and again.

So superworm became vulva varicositie instead, and it got to the point where there were three of us in the pregnancy: me, the baby, and her (because with a name like vulva varicositie she was most definitely a her). And the funny thing is a teeny tiny part of me even missed her when she disappeared shortly after the birth, never to be seen again. Presumably, she's still in there somewhere (it's a bit hard to tell under a four-times mum tum) but happily she decided not to make an appearance with baby number four. Which is just as well as there is *no way* I was going to break the internet by holding *that* up to the camera and showing my midwife over Zoom.

4. Queefing is an occupational hazard.

Yes, I *am* talking about fanny farts. Of all the things they don't tell you about childbirth, vaginal flatulence has to top the list as *the* most unexpected and horrifying occupational hazard. Or queefing as it's also known (which quite frankly has to be up there with vulva varicositie for The Best Name Ever when it comes to lady bits). Type 'fanny farts' into an internet search engine and the very first suggestion to come up is 'fanny farts postpartum', yet literally *no one* talks about it.

Of course, it's so obvious when you think about it: your foof has been stretched within an inch of its life so *of course* it's going to take a while to get back to its normal (or as normal as it's ever going to be) size again. Fanny farts are simply par for the course. But the trouble is, like a 'graze' being worse than a tear, you *don't* think about it.

Pre-kids queefing hadn't even occurred to me until a friend living in a four-floor townhouse with four flights of stairs revealed she queefed going *up* as well as down the stairs after the birth of her babies. I was horrified – and I've never been able to look at those stairs in the same way again since.

Luckily we live in a flat with a lift so I think I've had a lucky escape on the queefing front. A lockdown silver lining for us corona mamas has to be that we could queef in the comfort of our own homes, instead of accidentally in coffee shops or at post-natal yoga classes. And if it did accidentally happen in public (by which I mean the aforementioned supermarket queue, because during lockdown going to the supermarket is literally as good as being 'out out' got) it didn't matter because whether you were dying of embarrassment or laughing so hard you were about to wet yourself because you could hide behind your mask.

Because there's nothing funnier than a fanny fart. The only thing funnier than a fanny fart is someone else's fanny fart. And fanny fart stories. Like the one about four flights of stairs and four flights of fanny farts. We've dined out on that one for years, and I'm quite sure I'll laugh about it for the rest of my life. And now you can too. You're welcome.

5. The first wee and poo aren't as terrifying as they sound.

A bit like midwives armed with fishing nets, the thought of that first number one and the first number two after giving birth haunted me throughout my first pregnancy, to the point it became A Thing. But the thing is, it needn't be A Thing.

If you happen to be catheterised as far as number ones go you won't even know, because that bag you can't unsee hanging down the side of your bed will silently fill up like magic and you won't feel a thing. And if you haven't been catheterised you still might not know, because let's just say the hatch is open, if you know what I mean.

But all the talk of flood gates opening and 'gushing' in internet chatroom threads (the ones you know you shouldn't click on but simply can't resist even though it's a rabbit hole and you'll easily lose a few hours) really isn't as bad as it sounds. And even if it is, by the time you've actually had the baby you really won't care. Gushing is the least of your worries.

Of course, if you've had stitches you definitely *will* know when it comes to doing a number one because as we've already established it'll sting like a b*tch. Which is where weeing in the bath or shower and spritzing your bits comes in.

Then there's the first number two, or 'emptying your bowels' as they so eloquently put it. I spent the whole of my first pregnancy worrying about it, but by the time you've pushed a baby out it's yet another thing you suddenly don't care about anymore. Because nothing is as frightening as pushing something the size of a watermelon out of a hole the size of a grape, and once you've done that, you can do anything. Including a postpartum poo.

6. The best way to dry your lady bits afterwards is with a hair dryer.

And I don't just mean downstairs lady bits, I mean upstairs ones too. Like queefing, why does no one tell you this? I shudder to think how many towels I ruined and winces I caused in the weeks after baby number one when a hair dryer will do the job in half the time and with none of the pain.

Admittedly you look like a moron standing in the middle of the bedroom with your legs akimbo waving a hairdryer about your bits, but it's *far* preferable than trying to pat things dry with a towel, plus you won't ruin the towel. (Just don't let the hairdryer linger downstairs too long if you've had stitches though, because it turns out they heat up too. And yes that is as ouchy as it sounds).

If you're a breastfeeding or pumping mama a hairdryer is also far preferable for drying upstairs too, because in the early days even the softest, fluffiest towel will make your eyes water. Imagine rubbing sandpaper over your nips and you're there. (Again, don't let the hairdryer linger too long upstairs either though, because if you heat them up too nicely you're in danger of triggering the let-down reflex, which is a bit like a fire hydrant going off). Which brings us nicely onto another thing they don't tell you.

7. You'll feel like you're leaking from every orifice.

Forget tears running down your legs, milk will run down your legs too. And the red stuff. Essentially you *are* leaking from every orifice: upstairs, downstairs, and - if you're having a particularly bad day – from the eyes too.

The first few days of it are one thing when it's all new and you're too high on newborn hormones and oxytocin to care, but it's around the two-week mark that I've really had a sense of humour failure about it. When the days and nights blend into each other in the sleep-deprived fug of new motherhood and it feels like all you're doing is endlessly replacing soggy pads.

You think it'll never stop: when it comes to downstairs it's simply *impossible* to get from the bath or shower to a towel quick enough without painting the bathroom floor red along the way and upstairs is a bit like a hose you can't control. You hear the term leaky boob bandied about a lot, suggesting a sort of gentle dribble a bit like a slowly dripping tap. But the truth is they don't just leak and they don't just dribble. When they really get going they jettison milk in every possible direction. Their face, your face, and – if they happen to be sitting too closely – unsuspecting visitors' faces too.

Of course, spraying unsuspecting visitors with milk wasn't a problem in the middle of a pandemic because we didn't have any (visitors I mean, not milk). Literally no one came to visit us in the weeks and months after Violet was born because no one was allowed in – not even midwives and health visitors. And I'll be honest: it was marvellous.

There was no need to get up and dressed and look vaguely presentable because people were 'dropping by' to meet the baby; there was no racing around in a bra and thong with your hair in a towel kicking discarded pants and socks under beds and hiding dirty dishes in the oven when visitors decide to turn up unannounced; there was no getting up and down like a yoyo producing endless cups of tea for visitors who offer to do it themselves shortly before planting their bums on the sofa and forgetting all about it because they're holding the baby and, *best* of all, there was no-one to make well-meaning but unhelpful suggestions like 'have you tried sleeping when the baby sleeps' and 'aren't they sleeping through the night yet?'

It didn't matter if you were walking around with two wet patches from 'leaky' boobs on the front of your top, your nursing bra straps unclipped, a boob hanging out and sick on your shoulder because there was no one there to see it unless you include the cats, but they don't count. (Just remember that the postman though *does* count though, but more on him when we come to confessions from the lady with the boobs).

But back to the leaking, and thinking it will never stop. The funny thing is it stops as suddenly as it started, and you'll forget all about it, just like the birth itself. Until you do it all over again, and it all comes flooding back. If you'll excuse the pun.

8. Being padded up to the nines upstairs and downstairs is pants.

You might forget about leaking from every orifice, but you won't, however, forget that being padded up to the nines upstairs and downstairs is pants. Like the leaking, the sense of humour failure comes at around the two-week-endlessly-replacing-soggy-pads mark, and you not only wonder if it will ever end but can't remember a time when you weren't one giant walking pad.

And it's even more pants when you're trying to pack a hospital bag but can't get hold of said pads for love nor money. Just like loo roll and linguini, in the first lockdown, the nation was panic buying panty pads too - and for some unknown reason, the super-duper thick ones you especially need after giving birth were especially hard to get hold of.

As if the stress of giving birth in the middle of a global pandemic wasn't bad enough, I had to traipse around three different supermarkets to get my hands on just one pack of sanitary towels, which wasn't even going to last the first day. They were sold out *everywhere*, and a question that still bugs me, a bit like the flashing fuel light in confessions from the head end, is what on *earth* were people doing with them?

Emergency bandages? Draft excluders? Fire starters? An alternative to loo roll because all the loo roll was sold out too? Insoles because all the shoe shops were shut? The mind boggles.

Nappies were also on the stock piling list, *not* helped by the fact there was a video going around the internet about how to turn them into face masks. In the days before face masks became mandatory some bright spark worked out that by cutting a hole in a disposable nappy, putting it over your head, and taping the tabs over your ears you were left with a perfectly fitting, tailor-made face mask. I had to bite my tongue when I saw a woman actually wearing one in a supermarket that had sold out of the very nappies I needed for my hospital bag.

I did eventually manage to get my hands on the necessary pads, but only because our lockdown baby was nine days late which bought me more time. And I did manage to get my hands on the necessary nappies too, but only because family, friends, and complete strangers rallied round to help (I will be eternally grateful – you know who you are!)

Ironically given that pads and nappies were like gold dust, I ended up coming home from hospital with more pads and nappies than I went in with. And I wasn't the only one. Hospital PPE gear might have been in short supply at the start of the pandemic, but there was no shortage of pads and nappies. They were stacked up everywhere, and the midwives were giving them out (in hindsight and owing to the lack of PPE gear perhaps I should have shown them the nappy/facemask hack).

It wasn't only carers I clapped for at 8 o'clock that Thursday night with my newborn baby in my arms when hanging out of your living room window banging pots and pans for the NHS had not only become a perfectly rational thing to do but a highlight of the week. It was the midwives who sent me home with everything I needed on the lady bits front so I could concentrate on recovering from the birth and bonding with my baby, instead of worrying about where my next pack of pads was going to come from.

I was also grateful I didn't give birth during Wales's 'firebreak' lockdown later in the year when a certain well-known supermarket chain (let's just say every little *doesn't* help) temporarily banned the sale of sanitary towels because they claimed they were a 'non-essential' item. Try telling *that* to a ward full of mamas who have just given birth.

9. It's surprising how quickly you heal.

Even if you have to sit on a rubber ring for 10 days and even if you find yourself twanging in the wrong direction in the supermarket queue in Tesco. You may *feel* like you've been in a car crash with stitches in the last place in the world anyone would ever entertain having stitches, but it really is surprising how quickly you heal.

It all starts with that first bath, when you're back at home and clean and dry and in your own clothes and your own bed. The feeling is almost (but not quite!) as good as the tea and toast they give you after giving birth in the comfort stakes. A week or so after that you'll realise that the black bits floating around in the bath are, in fact, your stitches starting to dissolve, and a week or so after that, when you've *finally* been able to ditch the downstairs pads, you realise you're starting to feel vaguely human again even if you can't remember the last time you slept through the night.

Just don't forget to spritz your bits, dry them with a hair dryer and laugh about queefing. Because if you didn't laugh you'd cry. And don't look at the exit wound. Ever. Trust me. Don't even go there.

10. The 'new normal' is the same, but different.

I don't mean life after Covid, I mean our bodies after giving birth. A friend once told me that having two babies had devastated her body. English isn't her first language and I assumed she'd used the wrong word, but it turns out devastated is *exactly* what she meant.

Like pooing in childbirth I remember being really really *really* worried about what pregnancy would do to my body and what the 'new normal' would look like afterwards. Especially when you hear horror stories about devastated bodies, prolapsed wombs, and holes where there shouldn't be holes.

But like floating turds, postpartum poos, and so many other things, when it came down to it, it turns out I didn't care.

I don't care that I've been left with a belly button like a crater and a wonky linea nigra that won't disappear no matter how many magic creams I slap on it. I don't care that the skin on my upstairs lady bits resembles crepe paper after breastfeeding not one, not two but four different babies. And I don't even care as much as I thought I would that I've got a mum tum that I can't shift for love nor money (abs, it turns out, are *not* made in the kitchen). I don't care that my breasts now appear to have eaten themselves (which, it also turns out is an Actual Thing, but more on that when we come to boobing). They're my tiger stripes of motherhood, and I wear them with pride. (I am glad vulva varicositie disappeared though, as I'm not sure I'd wear her with pride).

I'm a bit rounder and a bit softer and a bit wonkier with one or two holes that are bigger than they were. And that's ok. After all, it would be strange if our bodies *didn't* change after growing a baby and pushing it out. Even if it means you've got to go up a size in tampons for fear of sneezing them out. No one can go through that sort of thing and come out unscathed. And it took me actually *doing* it to realise.

There was also one *big* lockdown silver lining on the lady bits front: thanks to Covid and not one, not two but three different lockdowns I was able to hide away for the best part of a year while getting to grips with my new normal. Even better, everyone else was embracing a new normal too because they couldn't do the things us mamas don't get to do in the first year because we don't have the time, the energy, or the inclination either. Like having your roots done, sneaking out for a mani, and booking a Brazilian. Baby or no baby, we were all in it together and forced to channel our inner earth mothers whether we liked it or not.

For the first time that crazy hormone-fuelled breastfeeding hair didn't look *quite* so crazy next to everyone else's crazy lockdown hair. My uneven and cack-handedly applied home dye job didn't look quite so uneven and cack-handed next to everyone else's uneven and cack-handedly applied home dye jobs. And my postpartum mum tum could (just about) be mistaken for a lockdown stone (or two) and legitimately hidden under loungewear, which like hanging out of your living room window banging pots and pans for the NHS had suddenly become perfectly acceptable during lockdown. And that, people, is what's known as a #mumwin.

"Wrestling your own tit from the jaws of a sleeping baby has to be up there with vulva varicosities and fanny farts when it comes to things they don't tell you"

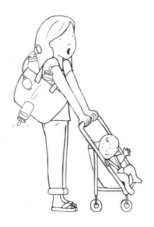

Chapter 3:
Breastfeeding

Confessions from the lady with the boobs: why I gave up my dream job to breastfeed, the day I made breast milk eyedrops, and circuit breaking the milk monster.

They say if you want something done ask a mum; I say if you want something done ask a *breastfeeding* mama. Because there's nothing a breastfeeding mama can't do. Superpowers, other than being the sole source of nutrition for a baby, include: becoming a queen of one-handed multi-tasking (although not necessarily in a good way); opening and closing things with your teeth and other body parts; sipping tea (or wine) over a wriggly baby's head without spilling it and getting your hands on objects which are *always* – no matter how much you plan for the next feed – inevitably *just* out of reach. All while surviving on the least sleep ever and being permanently bursting for a wee. Because you *always* need a wee the moment they decide to settle down for a feed.

I first started breastfeeding when Bluebell was born in August 2011, and at the time of writing, I've spent a combined seven years and counting with a baby on the boob. I didn't plan it that way - a bit like accidentally having a fourth baby, it just sort of happened. The truth is that once I'd started it was easier to carry on than it was to stop, so that's how I inadvertently found myself still breastfeeding after a year.

And there's *a lot* they don't tell you about that year (or in my case two, because that's how long it ended up taking to wean each of them off). Like the fact your angelic bundle of joy suddenly transforms into what can only be described as a piglet snuffling a truffle when your milk comes in, snorting and honking and grunting. And how they become conditioned to the sound of your nursing bra clip a bit like Pavlov's dog. And the fact there's a good chance you'll be left with a milk monster you created at the end of it.

So, after four babies - including an accidental lockdown one - here's what I wish I'd known about breastfeeding:

1. Fed is best.

When it comes to motherhood if there's one thing people get the *most* Judgy McJudgeface about it *has* to be feeding. Firstly whether you choose to do it by boob or by bottle, and later whether you choose to do it from a spoon or by popping - or dumping depending on which way you look at it - 'finger food' on a highchair and leaving them to it. (I'll give you three guesses which camp I fall into, but more on that when we come to weaning and confessions from the splash mat).

Literally everybody has an opinion about breastfeeding. And when I say everybody, I mean *everybody*. Even if they don't have breasts (in fact they can be the worst offenders). And they don't mind sharing it with you, either. But the fact is being a good mum isn't based on your ability to produce milk. A bit like what you got in your GCSEs or whether you passed your driving test the first time or *cough* the fourth time a few years down the line nobody asks (or cares) how you fed your baby. Because fed is best and they're alive, aren't they?

2. Breastfeeding doesn't 'come easily'.

Of all the exasperating expressions about motherhood that's the one I hate the most. Just because your milk comes in as it's supposed to; just because there's plenty of it; just because your baby knows exactly what to do and is putting on weight *doesn't* mean breastfeeding 'comes easily'. It means it comes naturally. But that doesn't make it easy. They're two completely different things and there's a *big* difference.

There's nothing easy about being the only person who can feed the baby. There's nothing easy about broken night after broken night after broken night with *no idea* when you'll get to sleep through the night again. There's nothing easy about getting through day after day after day of broken nights when you feel like you could sleep for ten thousand years. There's nothing easy about bleeding nipples and mastitis or pumping milk no matter how many of the latest gadgets you've got. And there's nothing easy about cluster feeding. It's a *big* commitment and one only another mama can know.

There's also nothing easy about being almost permanently unhinged. I don't mean mentally deranged (although what with the sleep deprivation it can feel that way, but more on that when we get to confessions of a mama already tired tomorrow). I mean literally unhinged. What with the cluster feeding and the burping and the doing things one-handed it's quite easy to find yourself walking around with a boob hanging out without even noticing. Even our postman doesn't bat an eyelid – he's seen it all before.

3. It's not just about milk.

First time mum me thought breastfeeding was *all* about the milk: how much there is (or isn't); whether it's foremilk or hindmilk (and does it even matter?); the quality of it (first time mum me actually googled whether a Big Mac would make my milk less nutritious – it doesn't) and how many antibodies are (or aren't) in it. But it turns out there's *so* much more to breastfeeding than that.

I thought I'd need dummies and comfort blankets and night lights and soothers and machines playing white noise but it turns out all I needed was a pair of boobs.

Four times mum me knows breastfeeding is also a stress soother, a tantrum tamer, a teething tranquiliser, and an accident anaesthetic - and sometimes for absolutely no reason at all: just because. And breastfeeding for those reasons is just as important as breastfeeding for hunger. Which makes breastfeeding the ultimate all-purpose parenting tool when you think about it. Or as I like to say: when in doubt, whip them out. You've got a secret weapon right there in your bra.

Breastfeeding is also a jolly good excuse for a sit or a lie-down, and getting out of things you'd rather not do, like wiping the bottom of a fournado shouting 'f-f-f-finished!' from the bathroom. And why not? There have got to be *some* perks to being up at two o'clock in the morning, four o'clock in the morning, and six o'clock in the morning Every. Single. Day. Even if not wiping a bottom is as good as it gets.

4. Whoever said there's no use crying over spilt milk is wrong.

They say there's no use crying over spilt milk - except there is when that milk is your own and it's taken half an hour to express one measly ounce of it. I know because I've been there, done it, and cried the hot tears of frustration that come with accidentally tipping over the few drops you *have* managed to get out.

Why don't they tell you that pumping can be so *hard*? And that the harder and crosser and more frustrated you get, the less milk comes out? Add pumping while balanced on a closed toilet seat hoping the battery on your pump doesn't run out and people aren't wondering what on earth you're doing in there because it sounds *a lot* like something else into the equation, and it's a wonder any of us pump at all.

5. I'd be forced to make some tough choices.

Like giving up my dream job to breastfeed. Even though it made my blood boil, and even though I knew I'd still be smarting about it years later (and I *am*). Max was just 12 weeks old when an opportunity came up for me to do shifts on the features desk of a national newspaper. A job pre-baby trainee reporter me would have described as my dream job, it couldn't have come at a worse time. The shifts were nine hours in an office a four-hour round trip away, but it was one day a week at weekends and I was sure I could make it work. Except I couldn't, because despite what they say, you can't have it all. Not when it comes to exclusively breastfeeding and your dream job, anyway.

It wasn't that the newspaper in question wasn't accommodating. The fact I needed breaks to pump milk was fine, there was a room for me to do it in (although I chose to do it in the loo because I didn't want to make a fuss) and I could even store my milk in the office fridge next to the actual milk.

The problem was (and is) that pumping at work is completely unsustainable. Because those 'breaks' to pump milk aren't in addition to lunch and coffee breaks, they're instead of. Meaning you don't get a break at all. And sitting on a closed toilet seat to pump milk as fast as you can knowing your colleagues are all hard at a different kind of work is not conducive to the relaxed atmosphere needed to empty a boob. Of course, getting stressed about the fact everyone else is working while you're not (except you are – you're busy being a one-woman milk machine) means it takes even longer than it otherwise might to get the necessary milk out.

As if that wasn't bad enough (and it *was*), spending all week trying to pump enough milk to leave while I was at work - and extra, just in case - while at the same time doing normal feeds was exhausting, stressful, and ultimately unworkable. How anyone manages to hold down a full-time job while exclusively breastfeeding is beyond me. Knowing Misery Guts was at home after his own working week trying to bottle feed pumped milk to a baby who didn't want to be bottle-fed didn't help on the mum guilt front, either.

So, somewhat inevitably and *very* grudgingly, after a couple of months, I finally conceded enough was enough. I didn't *need* this job; I wanted it. Which begged the question: who was I doing this for? The truth was I was doing it for me, but it wasn't about me, it was about my baby and our family. So I admitted defeat, handed in my notice, and wiped more hot tears of frustration from my face. Then I put my high heels and smart suit away, put my hair in a mum bun, changed into a pair of leggings, and went back to breastfeeding from the comfort of the sofa in front of Homes Under the Hammer while bursting for a wee with the remote control inevitably and (weirdly reassuringly) *just* out of reach.

Two more breastfed babies and a *very* stagnated career later I'm still smarting about it, but I don't regret it. Even though I know it's yet another example of the motherhood penalty and it makes me SO mad. Because it turns out being a mummy is a dream job too. Most of the time.

6. No one's looking.

You *think* they are, but they really aren't. And even if they are the chances are it's to offer you a smile or a nod of encouragement. You hear all sorts of horror stories about breastfeeding in public but in my seven years and counting of boobing, I've never once had a negative look or comment while breastfeeding out and about. (Or not to my face, anyway).

I have, however, been on the receiving end of some double takes and incredulous looks, but not because I was breastfeeding in public. Because I was breastfeeding a chest-thumping toddler. (Your chest I mean, not their own. Which is another thing they don't warn you about breastfeeding). No one bats an eyelid when you're nursing a newborn baby, but once they're a bit bigger it's a different story. Of course part of the problem is that, by then, muslins are useless. As are any other form of breastfeeding cover. They'll rip them off and fling them over the other side of the room before you can unclip your nursing bra. And you can't blame them − I wouldn't want to eat my lunch with a blanket over my head, either.

So while the great British public may not be looking (but might be if you happen to be feeding a chest-thumping toddler), by the time your little bundle of joy starts taking an interest in the big wide world around them they're most definitely looking. At everything while you're trying to feed them at the same time. Resulting in the unfortunate case of chewing gum boob, which can only be described as them turning their head to look at something − taking you with them. Think Elastigirl from The Incredibles and you're there.

The advent of chewing gum boob means your days of brexting and watching Homes Under the Hammer while nursing are numbered: instead you've got to put your phone down and the TV on mute in favour of sitting in total silence without making eye contact lest they get distracted and take you with them.

Boob to cot transfers are the worst, when you've successfully heaved yourself off the sofa using no hands because you've got a sleeping baby in your arms, stealthily made it to the bedroom and successfully laid them in their cot without waking them, only to stand up and find your boob still lodged firmly in their mouth. Apart from being yet another thing you can't unsee, wrestling your own tit from the jaws of a sleeping baby has to be up there with vulva varicosities and fanny farts when it comes to things they don't to tell you. Because if they did you'd think twice about having a baby in the first place.

7. There are some surprising uses for breastmilk.

I'm not talking about ice cream or cheese — that's just weird. I'm talking about eye drops and jewellery (which admittedly also sound weird, but bear with me). It turns out they call breast milk liquid gold for a reason — there's *all* sorts you can do with it. Aside from the aforementioned ice cream and cheese, which tend to make headlines for all the wrong reasons, there are also some *really* clever uses for breastmilk. Like clearing up blocked tear ducts, easing eczema flare-ups, and zapping eye infections. I know because I keep a sachet of it in the freezer between the peas and alphabites, just in case.

I first discovered the healing properties of breastmilk when the doctor told me there was nothing we could do about Max's blocked tear ducts other than keeping his eyes clean. He was only a few days old and his little eyes were so gummy they were sealed shut with gunk. Watching him trying – and failing – to open his eyes was more than three-days-postpartum Mama Bear me could cope with, so exasperated with the doctor and feeling powerless I did what they always say you shouldn't do and asked the internet. It was there that I found lots of other mamas declaring breastmilk the perfect, natural, magical remedy for gummy eyes and a host of other things since the dawn of time (apparently the beneficial bacteria in breast milk is also effective against certain strains of gonorrhoea, but let's not go there). Or the dawn of the world wide web anyway, which is 1989. I know.

So, weighing up the pros and cons of putting drops of breastmilk in my newborn baby's eyes (the pros being it might actually work, the cons being what could go wrong?) I decided to give it a go and try making breastmilk eyedrops. Not directly from boob to eye - mainly because I couldn't work out how that would work logistically - but by expressing milk first and dropping it into his eyes (I knew all those syringes that come with kids' medicine and end up jamming up the cutlery drawer would come in handy for something one day).

And do you know what? It actually worked. Within hours his eyes his gummy eyes were gunk-free and open and clear again like nothing had happened. A few months later I discovered breastmilk does an equally magic job on cracked nipples (mine I mean, not theirs) and fast forward two years and it also helped heal Marigold's outbreaks of eczema.

So, feeling smug with new-found self-doctoring skills, the last thing I've done before calling time on the milk bar with each baby is pop a big sachet of expressed milk in the freezer. When it comes to minor ailments my first port of call is always breastmilk. Even for the grown-ups. I've dropped it in eyes, poured it in ears, rubbed it on bottoms, and applied it to chicken pox and, in a bid to remember just how amazing breastmilk actually is, I've even had some of it turned into jewellery.

I know it's not everybody's cup of tea (or milk) but after everything my boobies have done – feeding four babies exclusively for the first six months of their lives and then for another 18 months each afterwards - encapsulating some of my breast milk in a piece of jewellery to keep forever seemed like the most natural thing in the world to do.

It was the thought of never breastfeeding again after Marigold was born that possessed me to do it. Grief might sound like a strong word to use, but that's how I felt in the days and weeks after giving up breastfeeding her because I thought she'd be my last baby. I genuinely felt like I was in mourning (very definitely a sign you're not 'done' mumming yet, but more on that when we get to confessions of an accidental mum of four). I asked the internet for help again, but there's very little about not wanting to stop breastfeeding and an *awful* lot on the jubilation and freedom of giving up.

So I set about finding someone who could immortalise my precious breastmilk in a piece of jewellery (you guessed it, I asked the internet again) and I'm now the proud owner of a little blue charm featuring six white breast milk roses (yes you did read that correctly – breast milk roses!) I love the fact that a little bit of the milk that fed my babies has been preserved in such a pretty way, and that only I (and now you) know what that bead around my neck is actually made of. In monetary terms, it's among the least intrinsically valuable items of jewellery I own, but in sentimental terms, it's absolutely priceless. And isn't keeping memories alive all any of us want to do?

8. There are also some surprising uses for boobs.

It's not just breastmilk there are surprising uses for. There are also some surprising uses for boobs. Like painting with them, which isn't as bonkers as it sounds. It's actually *really* liberating.

Whilst mourning the fact I would never breastfeed again after Marigold I was on a women's wellness retreat which included a boob printing workshop (we've got the Real Housewives of Cheshire to thank for a rise in popularity of those, apparently). Designed to promote body confidence and acceptance, boob printing is all about challenging the idea of what the 'perfect' pair of boobs should look like and empower women to celebrate theirs – imperfections and all.

The fog of grief must have got to me, because like breastmilk jewellery, painting with my boobies suddenly seemed like an *excellent* way to end and honour my breastfeeding journey.

Now, *obviously*, I'm not a real housewife of Cheshire – I'm just a knackered mum whose boobs have seen far better days – but I am immensely proud of the babies they have single-handedly fed and nourished. So I whipped off my top, painted a pink heart on each boob to represent the nurturing they have done, and printed them onto paper before going a bit mad with glitter in a room full of complete strangers I had never met before. And it was The. Best. Fun. Ever.

My boob art now hangs on the fridge next to paintings from nursery, gymnastics certificates, and PE kit reminders. It looks like just another piece of 'artwork' from nursery, and only we know it isn't. And now you, of course.

9. It's easier to carry on breastfeeding than it is to give up.

First time mum me thought establishing breastfeeding would be the hard bit, and stopping the easy bit. But what first time mum me *didn't* appreciate is that by the time I was ready to stop breastfeeding I'd have created a monster – a milk monster with absolutely no intention of giving up the boob.

Put 'breastfeeding at two' into an internet search engine and it will automatically predict you're searching for breastfeeding at two weeks or two months, not two years. I thought they'd self-wean, but they didn't. That's a big fat myth with bells on. The truth is my babies were as keen – if not keener – on the boob at two years old as they were at two months old. Leaving me with the unenviable task of circuit breaking a milk monster.

I had absolutely no idea how to go about weaning the strapping, chest-thumping toddlers in my arms. So I didn't. I just carried on and found myself extended breastfeeding (although I don't know why they call it that – it's just breastfeeding).

10. Milkin' it in a pandemic has its benefits.

Like not needing to worry who's looking, not needing to hide breast pads (a soggy one you tucked under a leg while feeding in a café but forgot about and spends the rest of your shopping trip stuck to your thigh is *not* a good look) and not getting as hangry as you would if you weren't in lockdown with *all* the snacks within easy reach.

Thanks to the pandemic and having no choice but to stay at home it was months before I breastfed Violet in public for the first time. There was no need to arrive somewhere you've never been before and do a mental reccy of the room before sitting down to work out where the best chair to nurse in is in case a random stranger sees a bit of side boob. There was no need to feel all sorts of weirdness when your boobs start leaking milk in response to a stranger's baby crying (thankfully my own family's Covid crying didn't have quite the same effect). And there was no need to get so hungry from running around doing the ten million things you used to do in a day before lockdown that you got so hangry you had a full-on mummy meltdown.

But *best* of all was free rein to live in breastfeeding-friendly loungewear, which had suddenly become perfectly acceptable attire whether breastfeeding or not. Everyone was wearing it, no matter what the occasion, the location, or what day of the week it was. (Which is just as well, because during lockdown most of the time I didn't have a clue what day of the week it was).

So, where previously you'd have to hunt down clothes that were suitable for breastfeeding in only to be forced to choose something you'd never normally dream of wearing if it wasn't for the fact you were boobing, suddenly there was an explosion in elasticated-waist onesies and wrap-front jumpsuits. Lockdown fashion was a breastfeeding mama's dream. (It turns out there is a *slight* occupational hazard with a jumpsuit though: you do need to make sure you know where the arms are when you're going for a wee. That's a top tip from a mama whose jumpsuit arms *might* have accidentally fallen in the loo while going for a wee once. Or possibly twice).

There was also no need to field silly and pointless comments from visitors who think they know better like 'she must be hungry' when she isn't and 'you're not feeding her to sleep are you?' when they know full well that's precisely what you're doing. At the time of writing I'm still at it with Violet, partly because it's easier to carry on than it is to stop like it was with the others, and partly because I'm absolutely terrified about what will happen when I do stop after reading something I shouldn't have done on the internet. (The internet's got *a lot* to answer for).

Apparently when a mama stops breastfeeding and her boobies go from being full-time milk machines to not being full-time milk machines the cells inside 'gobble up their dying neighbours'. That's what it actually said. Which basically means they eat themselves (according to the internet the scientific term is 'cellular suicide'). I don't know what happens after that because I stopped reading. The mind boggles and I don't want to know. What I *do* know is that the concept of boobs eating themselves gives a whole new meaning to the term fed is best though.

I also know that not all breasts are created equal. (I don't mean my breasts and someone else's – I mean my actual breasts). Because one of the things they fail to warn you about breastfeeding is that your previously equal-sized boobies can end up not being equal-sized owing to your little bundle of joy preferring one side to the other. The million-dollar question is whether my previously equal-sized boobies will return to their once equal size, or whether one will stay blown out of all proportion for the rest of eternity, but I still don't know the answer to that one.

If it turns out my boobs really *do* eat themselves and they don't return to their previously equal size I could always get a boob job, which is something I said I'd never do. But I didn't know boobs could eat themselves and be blown out of all proportion then. So never say never.

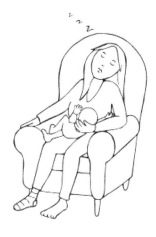

Chapter 4:
Sleep (or lack of it)

*Confessions of mama already tired tomorrow:
six in the bed, the big fat lie I tell health
visitors, and learning to live with outbreaks
of parps.*

Already tired tomorrow. That's how I feel most days and have done for the best part of the last 10 years. Which absolutely horrifies me when I think about it. So I do my best not to. Because parenting isn't nine to five – it's when you open your eyes to when you close your eyes (and quite a lot in between). Which makes for a *looong* day. And a bit like Brits being obsessed with talking about the weather, like many mamas I'm obsessed with talking about sleep. Mainly because I'm not getting any.

How much I did (or didn't) get last night. How ageing lack of sleep is (or isn't). How much the baby did (or didn't) get last night. How much Misery Guts *did* get last night (even though he claims he had a 'bad night' but I know he didn't because I was awake and he was snoring his head off). And how much my mummy friends didn't get either and where we all are on the 'which Ian Beale are you today' scale. (If you haven't seen it look it up – it's like the Britney Spears one, but funnier. You'll belly laugh, I promise).

And the thing about talking about sleep is that it means you can live (or sleep) vicariously through others. I love nothing better than hearing about someone else's sleep, *especially* if it involves a hotel stay or a mini-break. Because that's as good as it gets until they start sleeping through the night. And even then, if you're co-sleeping, it doesn't get much better.

As well as being already tired tomorrow, it wasn't until I became a mum that I fully understood what it means to be bone tired. Sometimes it feels like the only chance of catching up on the Lost Sleep of Motherhood is when I'm dead. (It also wasn't until I became a new mum on hijacked maternity leave in lockdown that I fully understood what it means to be at the end of your rope, but more on that when we come to homeschooling hell).

So, after four babies - including an accidental lockdown one - here's what I wish I'd known about sleep (or lack of it):

1. There are 10 stages of sleep deprivation.

Ranging from euphoria to being already tired tomorrow to total memory wipe-out. It all starts when you've been up for however many hours pushing a human being out of your lady bits. It's the hardest days' work you've ever done in your entire life, they're safe in your arms and you feel on top of the world and like you've *totally* got this. Then you surprise yourself with how little sleep you actually need (which is stage two). They might be feeding every few hours, it might be weeks since you had any meaningful sleep yet everything is going swimmingly. Perhaps Margaret Thatcher was right: four hours of sleep a night *is* all you need. Then comes stage three, when you realise she wasn't and it isn't. Because it turns out sleep deprivation is cumulative.

Stages four, five, and six involve waking up and

wondering how on *earth* you're going to get through the rest of the day, being unable to remember the last time you woke up and felt better, and being so tired you could weep. In that order. And you might have wept on the loo, or into (yet another) cup of cold tea. Even getting them dressed – never mind getting yourself dressed – seems like a gargantuan task. You totally *haven't* got this.

Then comes stage seven: total memory wipe-out. Like being somewhere you've been before and having absolutely no recollection of it. We were on a day out at a National Trust property once and I couldn't understand why Misery Guts was looking at me like I was mad when I commented on how nice it was and questioned why we hadn't visited before: it turns out we had but I couldn't remember a thing.

That's when being already tired tomorrow kicks in (stage eight), along with not being able to remember the last time you had a good night's sleep (stage nine). Finally comes the tenth stage of sleep deprivation: feeling like you could sleep for ten thousand years. You're perma-knackered and don't recognise the Gollum-like reflection staring back at you in the mirror. You know the old you must be in there somewhere, but don't have the energy to find her. If only you weren't so God. Damn. Tired.

2. Lack of sleep will turn you into a mombie.

Which is just like a zombie, but less bitey. It gets to the point, once you've reached the tenth stage of sleep deprivation when you basically feel like a dead person brought back to life. You unquestioningly and robotically go through the mundane motions of tying up nappy sacks and loading the washing machine without having any memory of actually doing it. Or the last time you brushed your hair. Signs you're turning into a mombie include: leaving the house and realising your skirt is on inside out (or, worse, that you're not actually wearing it at all); sitting up late in the evening, eyes stinging and body screaming for bed, just so you can have a bit of quiet, child-free time; and mumnesia: *completely* forgetting quite important things like half-term and why all the other kids at nursery are dressed as book characters and yours isn't. But don't dare question a mombie, or tell her that her skirt is on inside out. Because then she *might* get a bit bitey.

3. There are certain things you should never say to sleep-deprived mama.

Especially a locked-down, homeschooling one. Like 'you look tired' and 'have you tried sleeping when the baby sleeps?' The only thing worse than telling a sleep-deprived mama she looks tired is someone who isn't a sleep-deprived mama telling a sleep-deprived mama *they're* tired. No. No, you're not. You've got absolutely *no* idea.

But whether you're a lockdown-down homeschooling mum, a first time mum, a second time mum, or a veteran mum, there's absolutely *no point* telling a mama she looks tired. Because she already knows that. Instead, try telling her what a great job she's doing. Because she might not know *that*.

Then there's those who tell you their baby slept through the night at three weeks and those who tell you theirs didn't sleep through the night for three *years*. Both of whom are as bad as each other and deserve to have their heads banged together. Because not all babies sleep through the night. Especially breastfed ones.

They're also the type of people who will sagely go on to tell you 'it gets easier'. But the thing is, in the short term, it doesn't get easier. It gets worse.

Being woken up every few hours throughout the night is one thing when you're on maternity leave and all you have to do is keep everyone alive the next day, which can be done from the sofa wearing jim jams and without leaving the house. But it's quite another when life has returned to 'normal' and you're back at work and you're still being woken up every few hours throughout the night yet expected to function as an ordinary human being. It's even worse than when they were newborn. People think the days and weeks after the birth is when you need the most help and sleep and naps. It isn't. It's the days and weeks after that, and the days and weeks after that, and then the days and weeks after that.

While there are certain things you should never say to a sleep-deprived mama, there are also certain things you should never say to a sleep-deprived mama *in a pandemic*. Like 'have you seen this report about [insert coronavirus birth horror story here]' and 'what's the big deal - fifty years ago women gave birth without husbands or birth partners all the time!' That may be so, but that doesn't make it right. A husband or birth partner isn't just a visitor, they're an essential member of your birthing team. But pandemic or no pandemic, the truth is nothing you can say to a sleep-deprived mama is right. So don't say anything at all.

4. Lack of sleep can make you do funny things.

In addition to leaving the house and realising your skirt is either on inside out or you're not actually wearing it at all, lack of sleep can make you do funny things. Like getting the bus back from town only to get home and remember you drove there. And taking dirty towels on holiday with you because they've got a tumble drier and you haven't (although I'm still torn on whether that was, in fact, a genius idea or just plain stupid. All is revealed in confessions from the bottom of the dirty laundry basket).

Over the years funny things I've done through lack of sleep range from the stupid, like accidentally weeing on the dangly arms of jumpsuits even though I'd made a mental note *not* to accidentally wee on the dangly arms of jumpsuits, to the ridiculous: walking into a bank, arguing with the cashier about my account number only to realise I was in the wrong bank, to the really quite dangerous: picking the baby up in her grobag, walking around the room patting her back to sleep only to realise she was upside down and I was patting her legs not her back.

A retired midwife once told me that babies survive in spite of us, and I've always remembered that. Mine have *definitely* survived in spite of me and there's a jolly good reason sleep deprivation is used as a form of torture: it can make you go doolally.

5. There's tired. And then there's breastfeeding tired.

Breastfeeding tired is like pregnancy tired, only worse because it lasts for way longer than nine months. I thought the hardest thing about breastfeeding would be things like keeping up my milk supply and making sure the baby was getting enough milk. I didn't for one minute think it would be the tiredness.

Breastfeeding tired makes you do things like sit in the car outside your own house with a flask of tea because the baby is sleeping and you'll do *anything* not to wake her up (veteran mum me would have simply left her there and gone back to check every now and again). It's true what they say: if baby number one eats dirt you phone the doctor, if baby number two eats dirt you wash their mouth out, if baby number three eats dirt you wonder if you need to give them lunch.

Breastfeeding tired hits you between the eyes mid-afternoon and gets slowly but surely worse until you either succumb to a power nap (highly unlikely after baby number one) or push through with the help of one caffeine hit after another until you can collapse on the sofa with a glass of wine (highly likely after baby number two).

As a result of breastfeeding tired, you pick your battles, like letting them sleep beside you in the vain hope you'll be a little bit less breastfeeding tired.

6. Co-sleeping doesn't make you a bad parent.

.

And there's no need to feel reckless or guilty about doing it either (we put ourselves through enough as it is). Even doing it and then lying to people's faces about doing it doesn't make you a bad parent. And when I say people I mean quite important ones, like health visitors with clipboards who make disapproving noises. Because it turns out co-sleeping isn't necessarily a decision you make. Or not *your* decision anyway. It's one they make for you (your baby I mean, not the health visitor).

We've co-slept with all four of ours and still do with the younger ones (although technically you don't really co-sleep with toddlers - they sleep and you don't because the space they take up is *not* proportional to their size). Like extended breastfeeding, it wasn't something I deliberately set out to do, they just sneaked their way into our bed one at a time and before we knew it there were six in the bed and we all rolled over and the one who falls out is usually me.

It was easier to let them stay than it was (and is) to stop them, especially when they sidle in when you're sleeping and you wake up and they're magically there. And just like breastfeeding, *everyone* seems to have an opinion about co-sleeping, whether they do it or not. But the thing is co-sleeping isn't necessarily irresponsible and isn't necessarily dangerous, as long as you know what you're doing and you do it safely. It's the most natural thing in the world.

The fact was they slept best in my arms and next to me. And I slept best with them in my arms and next to me. The trouble starts if you have the misfortune of being allocated a midwife or health visitor who *doesn't* think they sleep best in your arms and next to you and doesn't think it's the most natural thing in the world.

Which is why not co-sleeping is a big fat lie I tell health visitors, the thinking being that what they don't know can't hurt them.

Interestingly, co-sleeping didn't seem to be an issue during the pandemic. I wasn't asked about it once. Which is a shame because telling the Big Fat Lie over Zoom with the help of a dodgy wifi connection would have been far easier than it is to someone's face. Presumably, they had more important things to worry about during the pandemic than who was sleeping where.

So, if co-sleeping is right for you (or if you can't be bothered to lie on a bedroom floor for two hours with your hands between the rung of a cot only for them to wake up the moment you try and crawl out like me) then arm yourself with all the facts and do it: co-sleeping doesn't make you a bad parent. At worst it makes you a lazy one. Although putting a towel over the wee spot and going back to sleep because you're so tired *might* make you a bad parent.

7. Kids smell.

Unfortunately, there's a lot more to co-sleeping than wee spots. Wee spots are the least of your worries. There are poo spots, chunder spots, bogey spots, and unidentifiable spots (it's best not to look too closely at those, and *definitely* don't sniff them). And then there are the parps. When it comes to co-sleeping, you have to learn to live with outbreaks of parps. Because it turns out kids fart. A lot. Trumps escape from their little bottoms all night long, to the point your bedroom sounds like a trumpet voluntary.

In fact, they're really disgusting creatures when you think about it. It all starts with the umbilical cord, which is another level revolting. Especially when it starts to fall off (why don't they tell you you're basically dealing with gangrene?) Why anyone keeps the stumps is beyond me. Then there are things like ear and chin cheese, which is basically sour milk going off behind their ears and in the folds of their creases. And as for toe and finger fluff – where on earth does *that* come from when they don't go anywhere or do anything? (Although I have to say extracting the lint from the crevices between their fingers and toes is *mightily* satisfying).

They also smell a lot (kids I mean, not their farts - although they do too). I don't mean that fleeting, amniotic, ovary-aching newborn smell you wish you could bottle. I mean after that. When their hair smells and their breath smells and their bum smells. And there's nothing worse than sleeping next to a smelly child breathing all over your face and coughing with abandon into your eyeballs all night long, even if it's your own.

So, if you're planning on co-sleeping my advice is this: buy the biggest bed you can find, and make sure it's got a footboard. That way you can use both ends. There's no such thing as too big. If I'd have known we'd routinely have all four kids in our bed at night we'd have gone for a super king, without question. We've even got one long bolster pillow so we can all sleep comfortably in a line instead of falling off individual pillows. Oh, and don't forget to open the window.

8. Competitive tiredness is an unavoidable parenting trap.

And it's a game you simply can't resist playing. Even though no one's sure what the rules are, no one enjoys playing it and there can't be a winner. It's simply irresistible.

You'd *think* you'd be too tired to argue about who's more tired. But no. If Misery Guts moans about being tired I simply can't help myself. I *have* to wade in with a mum snark. It's like a red rag to a bull. Because he sleeps all night, every night. And I don't. And sleep envy makes you do funny things. (If I wasn't so scared of knowing exactly how much sleep I'm not getting I'd get a fitness tracker, just to prove I'm getting less).

And the trouble with unavoidable parenting traps that you can't help falling into is that I find myself having imaginary conversations about them in my head, inner rage mounting until I'm in a mood but nobody knows why. Then before you know how you got there you find yourself competing for the title of most knackered. Which is ridiculous. There are no prizes for being the most knackered. (If there were *of course* I'd win them all. Hands down).

It's also impossible not to wade in with your own levels of exhaustion when a mummy friend shares with everyone what an awful few days they've had, and how they've never been more tired. Within minutes it's become a competition. There's *always* a little voice in my head that says 'you can't possibly be as tired as me'. Yet tiredness becomes all you can talk about. Who's had the most, who's had the least, how much you had last night, and how much you're likely to get tonight. Even though it's the most boring snoring subject on the planet and no one cares.

9. Bedside cribs are a game changer.

When I first became a mum a bedside crib was a novelty and the sort of thing you had to hire from the National Childbirth Trust for an exorbitant price, only to discover there was a waiting list as long as your pregnancy so by the time you actually got your hands on one they'd be six months old and it would be too late. But at some point between baby number one and baby number two bedside cribs became A Thing, and by the time baby number four arrived there were *at least* 10 different types to choose from and you could get them in the middle aisle at Aldi. Even in the middle of a global pandemic.

And the thing about bedside cribs is that they're a game changer when it comes to the night shift. Unlike a freestanding cot or a Moses basket, there's no need to leap out of bed for a heart-stopping moment because you can't see them breathing. You can just put your hand out on their little chest and feel it going up and down. There's no need to be up and down like a yo-yo all night picking them up for feeds, putting them down again, and resettling them. You can just slide them over, put them on the boob and then slide them back again. Breastfeeding and bedside cribs are the dream combination. And there's no need to fall out of bed when they've outgrown it and decided to sleep in yours because as well as a handy extension to a floordrobe a bedside crib also makes an excellent bum hammock.

Ours is still attached to our bed even though all the kids have outgrown it for that very reason: when left with the tiniest sliver of mattress to sleep on in a neck crickingly painful position I can curl up and park my bum in it so there's no need to fall out of bed.

10. There are actually some good things about broken nights.

No, I haven't gone round the twist with tiredness: there *are* actually some good things about being up in the middle of the night with a baby. Like full moons and sunrises you wouldn't see if you were sleeping. I had no idea the moon created actual shadows on our living room carpet until I became a mum. I remember seeing it for the first time and doing a double-take, thinking one of us had left a light on. In my sleep-deprived state, it took a while for me to realise the strange illumination was in fact moon beams. And it was *amazing*. The same goes for sunrises: without a doubt, some of the best sunrises I've seen are those I've happened to catch when stumbling about in the small hours dealing with a baby. Sunrises I simply wouldn't have seen had I been fast asleep.

There's also something super special about snuggling down with your baby when the rest of the world is sleeping. Even after four babies and goodness only knows how many hours lost to the Lost Sleep of Motherhood when they're big and grown that's something I know I'll look back on and wish I could do all over again. Even though I'm also so tired I could weep.

If there's one thing sleep (or lack of it) has taught me it's to be kind. Even if the sleep-deprived mama in question is in a mood and you don't know why. Because you never know how many times she got up last night. Even if you think you got up more.

"Motherhood is basically about wiping stuff"

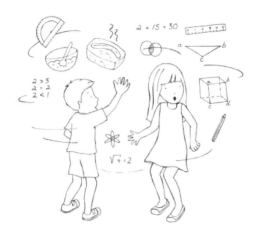

Chapter 5:
Homeschooling hell

Confessions of a (very) reluctant teacher: improper fractions, inner rage, and seesawing my way through a pandemic.

A bit like being a mama of four, if you'd told me I'd one day be a *homeschooling* mama of four, I'd have laughed so hard tears would not only have run down my legs but into my Ugg boots too.

Yet in March 2020, at 37 weeks pregnant and on what was *supposed* to be the first day of my long-awaited and highly anticipated final maternity leave (the one where I was going to do *all* the things I hadn't done with the others because you think you know better, like sleep when the baby sleeps) homeschooling is precisely what I found myself doing. Along with all the other unwitting parents of school-age children up and down the country (although knowing that didn't make it any better). I *thought* I'd been clever by taking maternity a week before the schools broke up for the Easter holidays so I had a week at home on my own before the baby arrived, but it turns out the joke was on me.

I suddenly found myself swapping maternity leave and tea and cake in coffee shops for home learning grids and banana bread I had to make myself, and just when I thought it couldn't get any worse, it did.

So, after four babies - including an accidental lockdown one - here's what I wish I'd known about homeschooling:

1. You need the patience of a saint.

And patience isn't one of my virtues. One of the things I very quickly discovered is that to homeschool you need *all* the patience, especially when it comes to accessing multiple online learning accounts on multiple devices with multiple passwords for multiple children with a husband on a short fuse.

Of course, what we were being told to do by the powers that be in their country piles with live-in nannies with absolutely *no* grasp of what it is they were asking us to do wasn't really homeschooling. It was remote learning, which is a completely different thing. Homeschooling is something you *choose* and make a conscious decision to do, with one timetable for the day and age-appropriate tasks for the kids involved. It's *not* something thrust upon you at zero notice and with no planning involving totally separate timetables that you do alongside other quite important things, like looking after smaller children and earning a living.

I also very quickly discovered (*much* to my surprise) that the school day is a *long* day. When they're actually *at* school the day goes by in a flash: one minute you're dropping them off, the next it's time to pick them up and you've barely had a chance to draw breath. But when they're at home and you're the teacher it's a completely different story. I counted down the minutes until home time every single day, except of course we were already at home.

2. Hell hath no fury like a woman scorned.

Or a mama expected to homeschool two kids of different ages while looking after a three-year-old and nursing a newborn baby. And little did I know just how bad it was going to get.

If we thought Lockdown 1 was bad, when they closed schools and nurseries with a few days' warning and sent the kids home with weekly home learning grids, Lockdown 3 was worse. This time we had less than 24 hours' notice and suddenly weekly home learning grids were replaced with daily timetables, pre-recorded lessons, and registration via Zoom because everyone except us had had nine months to prepare.

Swallowing down inner rage while simultaneously chiselling cheerios off the breakfast table to make desk space, trying to find the right Zoom codes, stop the printer from eating itself, and making sure no one was walking around naked became part of the morning routine. (I'm pretty sure an email from the school about appropriate dress code was directed at us). I hated Every. Single. Moment. And the situation was made even worse by the fact I *should* have been on maternity leave and snuggled up in bed smelling my newborn baby. I wasn't just a mama scorned; I was a mama incandescent with inner rage.

3. Seesaw is my own worst enemy.

That's what Max declared as we stared a new year and Lockdown 3 in the face, and I had to agree with him.

Seesaw was my own worst enemy too. If you haven't had the pleasure I'm not talking about the kind of seesaw you find in the park, I'm talking about a remote learning app that makes life *way* more complicated than it needs to be. I swear it was designed by someone who doesn't have kids. And if they do have kids they can't possibly have more than one.

It's almost as if they were trying to break us. Why does each child's account have to be accessed with separate login and password details? Why can't you simply have *one* account with multiple children in it, so you can flip between them instead of logging in and out ten million times a day? Why does everything you try and print out from it come out teeny weeny as though it's designed for a Borrower?

And then there was the stress of uploading work to it, which in many cases took longer than the work itself to complete. I don't think they could have found a less user-friendly system if they tried.

Thankfully there were some lockdown silver linings, even to Seesaw. Like workouts from the home gym of the kids' 20-something PE teacher, who gave Joe Wicks a run for his money and caused quite a stir in the class WhatsApp groups. I wouldn't be surprised if Mr Wicks saw a noticeable dip in viewing figures after that.

The truth is Seesaw is actually quite an apt name for it because that's exactly what I did: when it came to homeschooling I seesawed my way through the pandemic, bumping hard on my bottom on bad days and flying off my seat and high into the air on good days (although there weren't very many of those).

4. You need a degree in maths to teach maths.

Even to a six-year-old. Thanks to old maths versus new maths, even key stage one maths was beyond me. I found myself having to do the lessons myself first in order to understand the concept and then teach it to the kids.

Like Seesaw, they seem to have made maths *way* more complicated than it needs to be, with bases of ten and bus stop methods and mixed number fractions (I'm still not one hundred per cent certain what they are).

And as if old maths versus new maths wasn't bad enough (and it absolutely very definitely was), understanding the way things are taught now is like learning a whole new language. There are obscure anacronyms, like S2S (that's steps to success, in case you were wondering); 'spicy' English (that means a hard task as opposed to an easier one) and as for idiosyncrasies like fronted adverbials and split digraphs, don't get me started. The search engine and calculator on my phone have never had so much use.

5. Shielding myself from the class WhatsApp groups became essential to survival.

By which I mean muting them (I didn't have the guts to leave them altogether). Groups previously used to check if wellies were needed for Forest School and tongue in cheek 'which Britney are you today' quizzes quickly became a forum for conspiracy theories and dire predictions about the future.

On a bad day – of which there were many - there'd be 50 or more unread messages every time I looked at my phone. Threads ranged from questioning whether we were going to run out of wine thanks to the stockpiling preppers, to the desperate and bordering on hysterical proclaiming the world was going to end and we were all going to die. All of which was too much for a heavily pregnant, over hormonal mama stuck in a fourth-floor flat with three kids and no garden to escape to.

Even the mum whose sole reason for using the class WhatsApp group pre-Covid was to garner support for petitions against 5G phone masts joined in (her beef was with alleged radiation, not the spread of the virus, apparently). Funnily enough, she went noticeably quiet on the 5G front during the pandemic, when phones and mobile devices were her chief means of communication with the outside world.

The final straw came a few weeks into Lockdown 1 when the stay-at-home mums with huge back gardens, trampolines, *and* treehouses started moaning about running out of ways to entertain the kids. Of course, it was bad for all of us and we were all in the same storm, but it's true what they say: we weren't all in the same boat. Some of us were in yachts, some of us were in canoes, and some of us were drowning. I was drowning – and not just in a deluge of WhatsApp messages. I was sinking like a stone in a two-bedroom flat with no garden, four kids, two cats, and the aforementioned husband on a short fuse. So, I did what I should have done years ago: I muted the class WhatsApp groups, and they've been muted ever since.

6. Drinking on a school night (or day) also became essential to survival.

Lockdown 3 might have been worse than Lockdown 1 because schools had had time to plan and prepare for homeschooling and we were suddenly expected to deliver the same school day at home, but a lockdown silver lining was that I was no longer pregnant so at least I could self-medicate. By which I mean taking the edge off Seesaw with Sauvignon Blanc.

I shudder to think how many alcohol units we clocked up between Lockdown 1 and Lockdown 3 and how many times I was tempted to act on the advice of a meme doing the rounds at the time and simply stab a box of wine with a straw like a giant adult Capri Sun.

I knew things had got bad when I asked the Deliveroo driver delivering an emergency bottle of wine on a Tuesday afternoon whether he needed my date of birth as proof of ID, and he said no because he already knew it. Pre-Covid I would have been mortified, but somewhere between Lockdown 1 and Lockdown 3, I'd stopped caring.

I no longer cared about drinking on a school night (or day), and I didn't care about the increasingly frequent mid-week walks of shame to the recycling bin, either. This was a national emergency, after all. I didn't even care about getting caught drinking on the job, because who was going to sack me? You can't fire yourself.

7. You're not just a teacher.

Pre-Covid I thought being a stay-and-work-at-home mum was a juggle – and it *is* - but it's nothing compared to being a stay-and-work-at-home mum *and* a homeschooler.

You're the classroom assistant, the playground monitor, the dinner lady, the cleaner, the head teacher, the technical support, and the chief cook and bottle washer to name but a few. So you don't get a break at all.

What most people without school-age kids failed to realise is that we weren't 'just' homeschooling - we were setting lessons up, printing things out, clearing things away, producing *all* the snacks (of which there were zillions), refereeing playtime, making food, clearing it away and shouting (a lot).

Quite apart from being a mama with a newborn and outnumbered four to one, I felt like I was doing the job of at least five different people, and then I realised: I *was* doing the job of at least five different people. It was thankless, invisible, exhausting, and unsustainable, so when the Chancellor of the Exchequer had the audacity to 'thank mums' for juggling homeschooling with everything else I had a bit of a mummy meltdown in an incident involving alphabites. But more on all that later, when we come to confessions of a mama doing too many things and none of them well.

8. You can lead a horse to water but you can't make it drink.

Or in this case, a six-year-old to a computer logged into the dreaded Seesaw but you can't make it learn. While Bluebell (then nine) wanted to do all her homeschooling lessons and complete every task, it was a *totally* different story for Max who would whimper, whine and slouch across the table Jacob Rees-Mogg style. Every. Single. Day. To say it was painful – both for him and for me and for anyone unfortunate enough to be watching - is an understatement.

Unless it involved begging and bribery, trying to engage him in anything involving homeschooling was a battle, to the point we were essentially unschooling. And I don't blame him, because I wouldn't want me to teach me either.

At first, I took his refusal to engage personally and wondered what I was doing wrong, until I discovered some of his schoolmates had discovered how to use the chatroom function to type things like 'BOOOOORING!' in capital letters to each other during online lessons (top marks for spelling and punctuation – I'm not sure I could have managed that at six). The teachers were oblivious (it turns out they weren't *that* prepared, after all) and while I *ought* to have been cross, a teeny tiny part of me jumped for joy at the fact that, when it came to grasping the technology, they were as unwitting as I was. And like Seesaw being my own worst enemy, I was inclined to agree with the kids on this one too: remote learning *was* boring.

Staring at a screen was simply not the right learning environment for my reluctant pupil – he needed to be in a classroom with children of his own age and a teacher who actually knew what she was doing. Not in a learning environment run by an unqualified teacher with her baps out, a breastfed baby, an older sister crying over improper fractions, a younger sister watching Peppa Pig, and a dad shouting 'for fuck's sake' from another room every time it all got a bit much. Which was quite a lot. I think we can safely say that isn't a learning environment at all (unless you count Marigold repeating 'for fuck's sake'. In context. At nursery. Not my proudest moment). Which is where pandemic mum guilt comes in.

9. The only thing worse than mum guilt is pandemic mum guilt.

Of course, the fact that you worry about being a good mum means that you already are one, but that doesn't help when you've got two Seesaw accounts filling up with work there aren't enough hours in the day to complete, a baby who's decided to cluster feed and a washing mountain taller than you are.

Pandemic mum guilt, I quickly discovered, is just like normal mum guilt but with hurdles that weren't there when you started the race. Like phonics, improper fractions, and fronted adverbials. Pandemic mum guilt spread as rapidly as Covid-19 and by the time we got to Lockdown 3 I felt like a complete failure. Every. Single. Day. And I *was* - I failed at it spectacularly.

Because here's the thing: we're always told our best is enough, but during the pandemic, it wasn't. Every day the schools were closed the kids fell more and more behind because it simply wasn't possible for one person to deliver two completely separate sets of lessons to two children of different ages while looking after a baby and trying to work at the same time. What they were asking me to do was impossible.

All this came to a head when I got a phone call from school asking if we needed any help with technology owing to the kids' 'level of engagement', by which they meant lack of engagement. I told them in no uncertain terms it wasn't extra iPads we needed, it was an extra pair of hands – or three. This prompted what I'm sure was *meant* to be a well-meaning email saying they were sorry I was finding it so hard. But the way it was worded suggested I was the only one finding it hard and everyone else wasn't. That email exchange and what I *should* have said still rankles, in the same infuriating way as the flashing fuel light and recreating an argument with new and better points in confessions from the head end.

I *should* have said that I'd just had a baby and was supposed to be recovering from the birth. I *should* have said how many times I'd been up the night before – and the night before that, and the night before that. I *should* have said that breastfeeding a baby while trying to homeschool at the same time was quite literally back-breaking. I *should* have said that I needed to be on the sofa properly supported by cushions, not nursing one-handed at the kitchen table while navigating the vagaries of Seesaw. I *should* have said that I didn't ask for any of this and was just doing my best. And I *definitely* should have said that unless you've got the same number of children or more than me then don't question our 'level of engagement'. But I didn't. I laughed it off in the embarrassed way you laugh things off when you're put on the spot, and then I let even more pandemic mum guilt seep in.

It got to the point that I was so stressed out about the kids' 'level of engagement' that I'd upload anything to seesaw just to make it look like we'd done *something*. A tree climbed in the park (Forest School); making lunch (home ec); changing a nappy (life skills); getting mummy a white wine spritzer (hospitality). I felt like Big Brother was watching us and noting down all the things we hadn't done and would never do because there simply weren't enough hours in the day.

I could have cheerfully throttled every single one of *those* humblebragging mums on social media with their laminated lesson plans moaning about homeschooling yet proudly proclaiming they were 'done' every day at two o'clock, having ticked off everything on their super-duper lists. (We all know at least one).

By the time the kids went back to school after Lockdown 3 there were 51 outstanding activities in Bluebell's Seesaw account, and 48 in Max's. That's 99 lessons they haven't done and missed out on, partly because we'd had an accidental lockdown baby, partly because of the way it was delivered (the lessons I mean, not the baby), and mostly because I couldn't cope so simply gave up.

10. Giving a condom to a Beaver is a bad idea.

That's not a euphemism and I don't mean *that* sort of beaver. I mean a Beaver of the six-year-old, scouting variety. Unfortunately, it wasn't just school lessons that went virtual during lockdown, after school clubs like Brownies and Beavers did too. And, just like homeschooling, it was us unwitting parents who suddenly found ourselves thrust into the role of Brown Owl and Akela.

It started off straightforward enough with pen, paper, and felt pens among the items needed for each week's meeting. But by the end, I'd dread the weekly round-robin email of materials required because it meant either turning the house upside down to find one single split pin or braving the supermarket and risk catching Covid to try and get your hands on purple feathers and a unicorn horn when you couldn't even get loo roll or pasta. And you could put money on there being a great big mess to clear up afterwards too.

The longer lockdown went on, the more obscure the activities and lists of materials needed seemed to become as we all slowly but surely lost our minds. The cooking activities were the worst, involving things like armpit fudge (such a thing does indeed exist – more on that when we come to confessions of a mama at the end of her rope) and resulting in a kitchen floor stickier than a soft play café.

Activities at Crummy Mummy HQ included making kanelbullar (that's a Swedish cinnamon roll – I'd never heard of it either); constructing a lift out of a cereal packet and plastic straws (news of the ban on single-use plastic had yet to reach Brown Owl) and making a volcano out of a plastic bottle, bicarbonate of soda and food colouring (and yes letting six-year-old loose with food colouring *is* a very bad idea).

It all came to a head following an email with the words 'science fun!' optimistically typed into the subject line, which *of course* meant it was going to be anything but fun for the grown-ups. 'All' we needed for the planned experiment were three simple items: a balloon, sellotape, and a pin. Or they would have been simple, were we not in the middle of a global pandemic.

You'd *think* in a house with four kids we'd have the odd balloon knocking around at the back of a drawer, but after turning the flat upside down for the weekly 'pull random items out of my arse' mission for the umpteenth time it transpired not. So I sent Misery Guts to the supermarket to get some, but *of course* they didn't have any because there were more important things to stock in the middle of a plague, like food and water.

So Misery Guts sent me a message suggesting he buy condoms instead (when the notification flashed up on my phone for one fleeting, hopeful moment I thought he meant for us - albeit a year too late - then realised he meant for Beavers). And do you know what? For one horrible moment I *genuinely* considered blowing up a condom and giving it to a six-year-old Beaver for 'science fun'. That, people, is how loopy lockdown was slowly but surely sending us – and it would have given a whole new meaning to the term extracurricular activities.

"Suddenly using up manky old bananas seemed of vital importance"

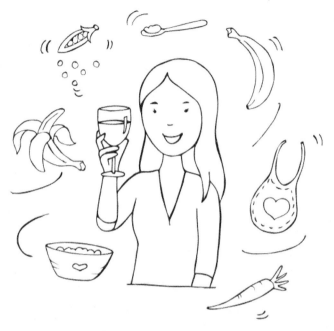

Chapter 6:
Weaning

Confessions from the splash mat: the real use for a peach baby food pouch, the mysterious case of the hoover and the haddock, and coping with a super spreader.

The thing about weaning is that it creeps up on you. You've *just* got breast or bottle feeding established, you've *just* settled nicely into a routine, you're *just* starting to think you've actually got this (whatever 'it' actually is), and then it's time to shake things up and start all over again.

You'd *think* four times mum me would know this – forewarned is forearmed and all that. But weaning has crept up behind me and bitten me on the bum Every. Single. Time. And every single time I've forgotten what a messy and thankless task it is.

I thought the terrible twos were the first tricky milestone we're supposed to face. It isn't. It's suddenly discovering you've got a tricky – and sticky – weanager on your hands. Signs they're a weanager include wearing more food than they actually eat and tipping everything onto the floor. Repeatedly. And they're only six months old.

The first time we went down the baby-led weaning route. The fourth time, when we were in the middle of a global pandemic with four kids at home, two of whom we were supposed to be homeschooling while the nation was panic buying fruit and veg, we didn't. Funnily enough, breaking broccoli into bite-size florets and boiling it (assuming you could get hold of it in the first place, that is) wasn't up there on my list of priorities.

So, after four babies - including an accidental lockdown one - here's what I wish I'd known about weaning:

1. Fed is best.

As we've already established in breastfeeding and confessions from the lady with the boobs when it comes to motherhood if there's *one* thing people get the most Judgy McJudgeface about it's feeding. Like breastfeeding, literally *everybody* has an opinion about weaning – and they don't mind sharing it with you, either.

First time mum me was sold on the baby-led weaning approach. Skipping spoon-feeding and pureeing everything within an inch of its life in favour of diving right in with finger food so they could feed themselves sounded *perfect*. On paper. *This* is what motherhood was going to be all about. I had found my calling.

Apron on and raring to do the job to the best of my ability, I embraced baby-led weaning with gusto. I peeled and sliced and chopped and grated and divided everything into tubs with labels and dates. Being so organised made me feel like the best mummy in the world. I'd *totally* got this (even though I still didn't know what 'it' actually was).

I bought heart-shaped tins for shepherd's pie, even though a six-month-old can't possibly appreciate a heart-shaped tin and there was no one else to appreciate my heart-shaped tins either because Instagram didn't exist yet. And I even screwed up sticky labels if I 'went wrong' when writing out what was inside my latest creation, starting again so it looked all neat and tidy. Then, in the evenings after Bluebell was in bed and with a glass of wine in hand, I'd open the freezer door just to look at all the tubs lined up and labelled. And do you know what? Seeing them all lined up in date order made me feel so happy. (If you're - quite rightly - thinking WTAF four times mum me doesn't recognise her, either).

There was something about cooking for a baby which seemed more important than cooking for anyone else, even though you very quickly discover the baby is the one least likely to be grateful.

But it turned out *this* was not what motherhood was going to be all about. I hadn't found my calling. Because baby-led weaning is all well and good when you've got a full year 'off' and only one baby. It's *not* so good when you haven't got a full year 'off' and you've got more than one baby. And it's *definitely* not good *at all* when you've got four at home and you're supposed to be home schooling in the middle of a global pandemic (although to be fair, all the food prep could technically be classed as home economics).

So we didn't do baby-led weaning the last time. It was shop-bought pouches all the way, with the odd alphabite or piece of pasta dropped on the floor by one of the others thrown in for good measure. Do I feel guilty about it? No. Ok, a bit. But just like the fact that being a good mum isn't based on your ability to produce milk, being a good mum isn't based on your ability to peel a grape or squeeze puree from a pouch, either. A few years down the line nobody asks (or cares) how you fed your baby - because fed is best and they're alive, aren't they?

2. Buying shop-bought baby food doesn't make you a bad mum.

First time mum me *thought* it did, but it doesn't. First time mum me inwardly curled her nose up at people whose idea of getting dinner ready involved reaching for a pouch – until I accidentally had a fourth baby in the middle of a plague and had to eat my words.

The fact is not only is shop-bought baby food more convenient, in many cases, it's better, cheaper, and more imaginative than anything I could peel or slice or chop or grate myself. The days of sugar and salt-laden jars are long gone and Violet eats things like organic Keralan curry and spinach masala. Things she'd probably take one look at and throw on the floor if I made myself. So why bother?

3. Baby food isn't just for babies.

There's *all sorts* you can do with it. Like transforming a glass of prosecco into a homemade bellini with the help of a peach fruit pouch. (For you obviously, not the baby. I'm pretty sure giving a baby a bellini is a no-no). And it doesn't stop there. A tropical fruit pouch will make a mean daiquiri, and an orange one will zhuzh up a mimosa nicely.

Baby food pouches also double up as an excellent pasta sauce in the same way stirring a can of soup through does (don't knock it until you've tried it). And the likes of sweetcorn hoops and parsnip puffs may have been designed for stage 2 weaning, but they go *rather* well with a nice cold beer or glass of wine. And even better they're less than 100 calories per bag – so positively virtuous too.

As well as opening up a whole new world of food I didn't know about, becoming a mum has also opened up a whole new world of food I'd totally forgotten about. Like fish finger sandwiches (now a work from home mum staple), alphabites (the fun to be had with those is endless), and kids' chocolate. Why *does* kids' chocolate taste so much better than normal chocolate? *Especially* when the chocolate in question is Easter egg chocolate? Surely it's the same thing? Is it the naughty treat feeling you get when you're eating it? These are the questions that go through my mind when I'm hiding in the kitchen cupboard biting the head off a Freddo frog.

4. Start weaning when you're ready.

Not when the books say you should, not when the label on the packet suggests you should, and *definitely* not when people who don't have kids say you should. Start weaning when you're ready and when they're ready (the day they start picking prawn cracker crumbs off the floor is probably a good indication).

It took four babies to realise that I should have trusted my instincts and gone with what's right for me and my baby right from the start, not everyone else who thinks they know better. At the time of writing Violet is still only on one meal a day and her main source of calories is still breastmilk. Because what's the rush?

The truth is weaning is a thankless task. When it comes to the invisible load of motherhood weaning has to be up there as one of *the* most invisible and thankless tasks. No one thanks you for the lost hours of planning and recipe researching and peeling and slicing and chopping and grating and cooking and portioning up and labelling. Not to mention the wiping. Least of all your baby.

I look at Bluebell and Violet now, one raised on homemade Kedgeree and Violet on shop-bought pouches and prawn cracker crumbs, and there doesn't seem to be any discernible difference between the two. They're both as fussy as each other and no doubt Violet will reach the terrible twos and refuse to eat anything except beige just like the others did too. So the longer you can put off this particular milestone, the better.

I'm also hoping that one day I'll get to watch *them* peel and slice and chop and grate vegetables for *their* babies only for them to take one look at it and throw it on the floor. And I'll laugh so hard tears will run down my face and into the white wine spritzer I'll be holding while watching fondly and reminiscing from the sofa.

5. Vacuuming up discarded finger food is a bad idea.

Especially if that discarded food happens to be fish.

One of the dishes peeling and slicing and chopping and grating mum me used to make was Kedgeree. Kedgeree was (and probably still is – I wouldn't know) a baby-led weaning mum's dream: perfectly balanced with protein (egg), good fat (haddock), and dietary fibre (peas). They can pick it up with their fists, swoosh it about the highchair a bit and the chances are some of it will make it into their little tummies.

The chances are rather a lot of it will also make it onto the floor, which in our house resulted in the mysterious case of the hoover and the haddock. It all started innocently enough: I'd lovingly prepared said Kedgeree and it was Misery Guts' job to feed it to the baby. I didn't think twice when I got home from wherever it was I'd been until there was a strange smell coming from the cupboard under the stairs.

After a process of elimination (it wasn't a dead mouse/ forgotten gym kit/discarded nappy) it was only when I got the vacuum cleaner out to use it next that I realised Misery Guts had hoovered up the haddock. And he hadn't emptied the drum afterwards. And now there was week-old haddock growing its own eco system in our vacuum cleaner.

Needless to say, we had to replace the vacuum cleaner (at the time I could have quite cheerfully replaced

Misery Guts too). There was *no* comeback from that. It's probably still stinking out a landfill somewhere leaving everyone nearby wondering what on earth the terrible smell is.

6. I'd rather starve than eat with my kids.

I'm sorry but it's true. Pre-kids I pictured sitting down around a table eating family meals together, sharing what we'd all done that day, and laughing happily. What I *didn't* appreciate is that eating with kids is like being the only non-chimp at a chimpanzee's tea party. And at the age mine are now I'd rather starve than eat with the kids.

I want to sit down at the end of each day with a nice plate of food and relax. But there's nothing relaxing, edifying, or life-affirming about eating with my kids. (Ask anyone who's had the misfortune of sitting next to us in a restaurant, but more on that when we come to turning into THAT family and confessions of a mama determined to have a nice time).

And when I say a chimpanzee's tea party, I mean chimpanzees with no table manners. How *on earth* can a baby project yoghurt far enough to make it drip from the ceiling? When did it become possible to ruin someone's day by having the audacity to put 'green' on their plate? Why does a baby throwing perfectly good food I've cooked from scratch make me want to kill someone? Why *do* they insist on reforming anything potato-based by rolling it into a ball in the palm of their hands before putting it in their mouth? And how hard can it possibly be to learn to use a knife and fork?

As a result, we rarely sit down and eat together as a family. Christmas and Easter are as far as I'll stretch. And each time I'm inwardly thankful we only have to do it once or twice a year.

So until the time comes when they can feed themselves without chucking most of it on the floor, rolling it into balls first, and/or catapulting yoghurt at the ceiling I'd rather cook two separate meals a day – one for them and one for us. Or starve.

7. Motherhood is basically about wiping stuff.

Why don't they warn you about the wiping? Endless, pointless-because-it'll-all-need-doing-again-in-a-few-hours-anyway, soul-destroying wiping. At least when it comes to things like breastfeeding and nappy changing there's an end in sight, but when it comes to wiping there is no end. You'll be wiping forever. Bums, floors, faces, noses, walls, wheels: you name it, you'll wipe it.

Admittedly having done baby-led weaning the first three times I only had myself to blame. If you think weaning is a messy business, baby-led weaning is off the scale. Food gets *everywhere*: in their hair, in their ears, in their eyes, up their noses, down their fronts, and even in their nappies. And ditto for you (but hopefully not the nappy, unless you've been particularly unlucky in the lady bits department). As for the house, mysterious crusts form on and in everything from lampshades to typically hard-to-reach places like button-back furniture, just to keep you on your toes on the wiping front.

It helps to invest in a highchair with the least amount of crevices. Our trusty Ikea Antilop bought second hand on eBay is still going strong after four babies and eight years and counting of being stood in the bath and hosed down with the shower extension (anything to get out of wiping).

And when I say food gets everywhere, I mean absolutely *everywhere*. Despite having cleaned the highchair down before storing it in the garage between babies I once discovered maggots living in the hollow legs. A whole collacine of them (that's the collective name for maggots, apparently). God knows how long they'd been there, and I'll give you three guesses what I did. I wiped them off.

8. Food (and toys) can change the colour of their poo.

I remember being at an NCT class and being shown a card with pictures of lots of different types of baby poo on it. There were black sticky ones, runny yellow ones, and hard round ones. What they failed to tell me about were bright green ones. And ones streaked with mysterious red stuff. And ones featuring pieces of Lego.

Because it turns out that blue bubble gum ice cream can turn their poo bright green. And it's so disturbing that they should really consider adding hulk poo to the NCT poo card (not that I've ever actually seen hulk poo, but it's what I'd imagine hulk poo to look like). It also turns out that sucking the head of a cuddly Elmo toy will result in poo with red fluff in it (and no there isn't any need to panic and call the doctor). And that pieces of Lego will go straight through them (thank goodness).

9. I'll never make banana bread again.

Just the smell of banana bread is enough to bring me out in a cold sweat. Which is a shame, because pre-Covid I actually quite liked banana bread. Post-Covid the smell of it makes me think something bad is going to happen. Like another lockdown, or worse: homeschooling.

Like sourdough starters and kitchen discos, banana bread went from having a moment at the start of the pandemic to becoming a middle-class lockdown cliché. And we *were* that cliché.

As news reports came in of panic buyers clearing supermarket shelves of household essentials and with UK borders closed suddenly using up manky old bananas seemed of vital importance. We couldn't *possibly* throw them away, even though flour was hard to get hold of too, meaning you had to buy the expensive stuff instead of the basic stuff. There were so many other things we could – and *should* – have been doing, like homeschooling, but there we were in the kitchen baking banana bread like our lives depended on it. The truth is, when I think back to that time, what we were doing is procrastibaking.

We developed several different variations of banana bread while we were procrastibaking too: we added almond flavouring to it (which actually tastes nicer than it sounds); we put lemon icing on it (Bluebell's idea – Bake Off has *a lot* to answer for) and we threw every sprinkle we had in the kitchen cupboard at it (and a lot on the floor).

We also spent a whole morning doing a 'stock take' of the kitchen cupboards after the extent of the nation's stock piling was revealed in alarming newsflash after alarming newsflash. This also suddenly seemed of vital importance, plus it surely classed as a lesson in household management (if I had £1 for every time I said 'not all classrooms have four walls' during lockdown I'd be *very* rich indeed). Instead, it turned into a lesson in what we *didn't* have. Instead of useful store cupboard staples like rice and pasta, we had ice cream wafers three years past their use-by date, *lots* of sprinkles, and Easter chick decorations for a cake we'd never made and probably never will.

The inventory is still stuck to the inside of the kitchen cupboard, written in an unhelpfully illegible orange highlighter pen by Bluebell (then eight). It includes things like coconut oil (another middle-class cliché, I know) and a packet of mint humbugs, neither of which would have been much use if the supermarket home delivery man really *had* stopped getting through or rationing was introduced. (Although to be fair there's a *lot* to be said for a mint humbug).

Each week I'd add packets of super noodles to the online Big Shop 'just in case' – even though no-one really likes super noodles and they used up two of our 85 rationed items per shop. To 37-week-about-to-give-birth-in-the-middle-of-a-global-pandemic-me it just seemed like a sensible thing to do. It still irks me that we were only allowed 85 items per shop too, regardless of whether you were a family of six like us or a couple of two. As lockdown went on it took me *ages* to get our Big Shop down to 85 items each week, agonising over whether choosing a bottle of wine over orange squash made me a bad mum. (There were some plus sides though, like the discovery of large-size cucumbers as opposed to normal size ones. And just how much wine you actually get in a box as opposed to a bottle. Who knew?)

As a result, I'd go as far as to say I'll never make banana bread again. A bit like using Seesaw after the pandemic (see confessions of a corona mummy and surviving a global pandemic) just the thought of refereeing the making of banana bread is enough to induce a post-traumatic stress-style twitch. Thanks to Covid, simple pleasures like biting into a freshly baked slice of banana bread have been ruined forever.

10. Weaning in a pandemic was an unexpected joy.

I know. I wouldn't put the words weaning and joy in the same sentence, either. But compared to weaning in real life, weaning in a pandemic turned out to be an unexpected joy. There was no need to plan outings around mealtimes because there were no outings. There was no need to plan for outings that *included* mealtimes because there were no outings that included mealtimes. (Unless you count buying a sandwich in the supermarket and eating it in the car, which I did once or twice just to eat something I hadn't had to make myself uninterrupted and in peace and quiet. But I'm pretty sure that doesn't count as eating out.)

There was no need to pack a nappy bag full of on-the-go snacks using all the Tupperware in the cupboard because we didn't even need a nappy bag. And *best* of all there was no need to get on your hands and knees and do a full deep clean of grotty coffee shop highchairs and their trays before you've even sat down and had a sip of tea.

Like breastfeeding and sleep, there was also no one to make silly and pointless comments about how you were (or weren't) going about it. There was no one to judge my shop-bought baby food pouches and the fact I'd left it until seven months before introducing solids because I'd been a *bit* busy trying to do the job of at least five different people.

So while weaning has crept up behind me and bitten me on the bum Every. Single. Time. (and every single time I've forgotten what a messy and thankless task it is) doing it in the middle of a global pandemic wasn't actually all that bad. Especially with a kitchen disco in full swing and a baby food bellini in hand.

"There's a pant cemetery at the bottom of our dirty laundry basket"

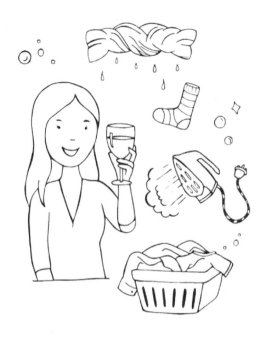

Chapter 7:
Death by laundry

Confessions from the bottom of the dirty laundry basket: where pants go to die, embracing the washing mountain, and why there's absolutely no point trying to flatten the curve.

Shortly after I announced I was expecting baby number three a friend, also a mama of three, told me I'd never see the bottom of our dirty laundry basket again. And she was absolutely right. I haven't seen the bottom of our dirty laundry basket again – not for years, in fact. I have absolutely *no idea* what's lurking down there. And I shudder to think.

Washing isn't really something they touch on at antenatal classes or in parenting books before you have a baby. In fact, I don't think I thought about washing at all. Which is perhaps why the volume and monotony of it came as such a shock. Just like co-sleeping and the amount of space a child takes up in bed, it turns out the amount of washing they generate is not proportional to their size. In fact the smaller they are, the more they seem to produce. Our washing machine is always on (and if it isn't, it should be).

So, after four babies - including an accidental lockdown one - here's what I wish I'd known about washing:

1. It's impossible to keep on top of the washing mountain.

Unless you've got two washers and two driers, a housekeeper or a baby that can do their own. Or all three. Washing is never-ending, and the sooner you get used to it, the better. Not only have I not seen the bottom of our dirty laundry basket for years, it's so rammed full we can no longer put anything in it either. As a family of six, we now have so much dirty laundry it resides in a permanent pile next to the dirty laundry basket, a washing mountain that grows bigger by the day. On some days it's taller than me (that's five foot six, in case you were wondering).

It's especially impossible to keep on top of it if you live in a flat with no garden and don't have a tumble drier. It takes a full 24 hours to get one load of washing clean and dry before you can put the next load on in our house, and despite the machine going on every single day, there's always a washing mountain. Add weaning and potty training into the equation and it's simply *impossible* to keep on top of.

2. The washing mountain can make you do funny things.

Like take dirty towels and sheets on holiday with you because they've got a launderette with industrial-size washers and tumble driers and you haven't. In the sleep-deprived fug of new motherhood after Marigold was born that's what I did on our first holiday as a family of five to a holiday park in Devon. And I was *mightily* pleased with myself for hitting on the idea, too.

At home, it would take three separate washes and three days to get all the towels and bed sheets washed and dried. And because we were going on holiday, there was no one there to do them so they'd spend our whole holiday teetering on top of the washing mountain smelling of damp waiting to be dealt with when we got back.

But with the help of industrial-size washers and tumble driers it would take just a few hours to get all the towels and bed sheets washed and dried, and they *wouldn't* spend our whole holiday teetering on top of the washing mountain smelling of damp waiting to be dealt with when we got back. So I packed them into a bag and put them in the back of the car next to the swimming towels and buckets and spades. It made *perfect* sense.

Four times mum me, who hasn't had a proper holiday since the holiday I spent washing and drying towels and bed sheets, wonders what *on earth* I could have been thinking. Who takes their dirty laundry with them on holiday? I should have been playing with the kids in the sand or simply sitting down doing nothing, not standing in a launderette on a holiday park feeling smug for folding hot towels.

It was around the same time that I started hanging out wet washing in the middle of the night. Not washing I'd planned to hang out, washing I'd forgotten about and suddenly remembered in the middle of a night feed when you start thinking about things even though you know you shouldn't. Because if I didn't hang the washing out there and then it wouldn't be dry by the next day, and then we'd be a day behind with the washing and then the washing mountain would get even bigger. So I'd finish the night feed, creep out of the bedroom, pull the wet washing out of the machine, and hang it out by the light of the moon, like a lunatic.

But as we've already established in confessions of a mama already tired tomorrow, sleep deprivation – and washing mountains – can make you do funny things.

3. The sooner you embrace the washing mountain, the better.

Because there's absolutely no point trying to flatten the curve. The fact is you've just got to learn to live with it (just remember to remove the skid-marked inside-out pants stuck inside inside out trousers from the top of the pile though, because no one wants to look at those).

Of course, you *could* get a bigger dirty laundry basket – or one for each bedroom – but that's not solving the problem, it's simply spreading it about a bit. And spreading it about a bit isn't going to make it go away.

So my advice is this: invest in holdalls. The bigger the holdall better. You can use them to hide washing; you can use them to transport washing; you can use them to do washing on holiday and if the washing mountain all gets a bit much you can climb inside yourself and hide from it.

4. The washing mountain has forced me to make some tough decisions.

Like how much poo on jeans is too much. (I don't mean my poo, I mean baby poo). And how many times school uniforms can legitimately be extracted from the dirty laundry basket, febreezed, and worn again.

The baby poo one is a tough one. How much poo on your jeans *is* too much? Does a *tiny* smidge from a nappy you quickly changed on the hall floor because they decided to fill it just as you were on your way out of the door and you're already late really count? If you can wipe it off with a baby wipe surely there's no need to add to the washing mountain – and make yourself even later - by going for a complete trouser change, *is* there? The same goes for goop and snot. If you can wipe it off with a baby wipe surely there's no need for an entire outfit change.

As for febreezing school uniform, unless you're one

of *those* mums with a separate set of uniform for every day of the week fishing jumpers and trousers out of the dirty laundry basket to febreeze them is simply par for the course. (Unless it's fish and chip Friday when baked beans are also on the menu, most of which they come home wearing and no amount of Febreeze will shift. But that's ok because it's Friday).

We also don't have any washing baskets (I don't mean dirty laundry baskets – we definitely have one of *those* – I mean plastic ones for clean washing). Because if we did it would be a case of 60 minutes to wash the clothes, 24 hours to dry them and up to a year to fold them and put them away. They'd probably never make it back to where they came from, and if they did the chances are they'd be outgrown. So clothes in our house go straight from the clothes horse to cupboards and drawers. Sometimes via a heap on the day bed in the corner of the living room.

5. Expect 'presents' from nursery.

When I say presents I mean presents in the *loosest* possible sense of the word. I don't mean 'artwork' or things made out of egg boxes. I mean neatly tied up nappy sacks of soiled clothes which they come bounding out of nursery merrily swinging from their little fingers.

At best they contain wet and dirty clothes from playing in the mud kitchen; at worst they contain accidental number ones and number twos.

These presents can range from one a week if you're lucky to one or two a day when you're potty training, and more often than not end up flung into (or at depending on the current height of the washing mountain) the dirty laundry basket to be dealt with at a later date. Then you find them at the bottom of the dirty laundry basket sometime later, stiff and dried and in some cases rock hard. The only saving grace is that you can't smell them, because *nothing* overrides the fragrance they douse nappy sacks in. And for very good reason.

As a result, there's a pant cemetery at the bottom of our dirty laundry basket. Along with a few socks and the odd pair of tights. Thanks to 'presents' from nursery, the bottom of our dirty laundry basket has basically become the place where pants go to die. Because of course they don't get dealt with at a later date. They stay there until the nappy sack itself has become stiff and dried and fossilised, and then you daren't open it so you throw it away. Which is what you should have done in the first place.

I'm pretty sure the 'gentle' reminders from school and nursery about bringing in spare sets of clothes are always aimed at me. What they don't seem to appreciate is that I've *deliberately* forgotten. Because more clothes = more washing. I'd far rather they came home from nursery in one filthy mud and paint-splattered outfit than with one filthy mud and paint-splattered outfit divided up into several neatly tied nappy sacks and wearing a clean outfit. Because we all know where the filthy mud and paint-splattered outfit divided up into several neatly tied nappy sacks will end up.

6. Because of the washing mountain I've got a dirty secret.

It involves dirty laundry (*lots* of it), twenty quid, and a man with a knowing smile called Stuart. Every few weeks I phone him up, pass him a holdall of dirty pants and socks, slip him twenty quid, and a few hours later he brings it all back washed, dried, and folded. Like magic.

Not long after Marigold was born it got to the point that our washing mountain was so big that an industrial-scale solution was needed, the sort of industrial-scale solution you'll only find in a launderette. What we needed, I realised when you start thinking about things even though you know you shouldn't in the middle of a night feed, was a *service* wash (looking back I'm not *quite* sure why it took me so long to hit on the idea, but it did).

So I phoned up the launderette and discovered the washing mountain that would have taken me five whole days to process and almost cost me my sanity could be dealt with by Stuart in three hours for twenty quid. And in my book that's twenty quid *jolly* well spent.

An added bonus was that there'd be no more crunchy crotches owing to Misery Guts not shaking out wet knickers properly before hanging them out. Because there's *nothing* worse than a crunchy crotch. (No matter how many times I tell him, he still doesn't seem to get it).

So now there are three people in our marriage: me, Misery Guts and Stuart. Every few weeks, when the washing mountain becomes insurmountable, we phone him up and he appears like a knight in shining armour and takes away all our dirty washing. Even in the middle of a global pandemic, when − mercifully - launderettes were classed as an essential service. Which is just as well, as otherwise, it would have been a case of death by laundry in our house. That or homeschooling.

It's not a case of can't be arsed, won't be arsed; it's a case of can't cope, send help. Leaflets for launderettes and service washes should be included in the information packs they give you in hospital: not pamphlets for newborn photographers and baby swimming lessons.

Stuart might be a dirty secret and the third person in our marriage, but he's a superhero I can't live without. The truth is he's one of the best things that's happened to us. Everyone needs a Stuart in their life.

7. Life is too short to iron.

Especially when you can buy non-iron school uniforms. And non-iron bedding. I simply don't understand people who can spend hours standing at an ironing board and actually set aside time to do it. They are *not* my tribe. And if you're one of those people with a giant steamer iron with its own docking station then I'm afraid we can't be friends.

I blame the fact I'm a forces child. Because there's ironing, and then there's military ironing. As a child ironing in our house involved starch and bars of soap and military creases for my dad's uniform, and if it wasn't done properly it had to be done again. There was level one to three on the iron and then there was Afghanistan level.

My mum (quite rightly) washed her hands of it and didn't get involved – I don't ever remember seeing her stood at an ironing board, and I don't blame her. What a royal waste of time. My dad did his ironing himself, handlebar moustache furrowed in concentration making sure his uniform would pass inspection (there was a uniform inspection sheet and everything). To this day he loves ironing. He'll sit in front of the rugby with the ironing board adjusted to the right level and iron away to his heart's content. Even tea towels. I don't get it at all. Life is too short to iron.

So those were my role models: a mother who refused to get involved with the ironing and a father who ironed as if his life depended on it (to be fair, in hindsight, it probably did). As a result, it's probably not surprising I've washed my hands of it too and don't get involved either. We do own an iron and an ironing board, but they don't get an airing very often. The dial on the iron broke sometime in the noughties so it's stuck on one temperature, and I've got no idea what that temperature is. I *do* know it's not Afghanistan level though.

Our ironing board came out one day during lockdown and Max (six) asked what it was. He thought it was a surfboard and it was a revelation to him when I explained what it was. He thought it was the best thing he'd never seen before. On the rare occasions the iron and ironing board do make an appearance I tend to only iron the bits you can see, like collars and cuffs. Because kids crease everything within five seconds of wearing it anyway. Before you've even left the house. So what's the point?

In my opinion, by far the best use for an ironing board is as a present wrapping station. With four kids ours has certainly been used more for that than it has for ironing. You can unroll your wrapping paper over either side without it creasing, you can stand your glass of wine on the bit you're meant to put the iron, you can line your pieces of sticky tape up next to it and little people and cats can't reach, rip or tear the paper before you've had a chance to stick it all together. Which is my kind of life hack.

8. Not washing bed sheets once a week doesn't make you a dirty b*itch.

Or a lazy mum. Three times mum me used to strip all the sheets in the house religiously once a week. Even if we'd been away for the weekend meaning they'd only really been slept in for five nights, at best. Every Friday morning without fail I'd wrestle with sheets, bang my head on the bunk bed and break into a sweat taking bedding off and putting fresh bedding on again. And as we've already established in funny things the washing mountain makes you do, I even took washing away on holiday to try and keep on top of it all. Because you wash bedding once a week, right? That's just what you do. Or so I *thought.*

At the same time I was religiously stripping (sheets) once a week, all the kids were sleeping in our bed (the gory details of which are revealed in confessions of a mama already tired tomorrow). It got to the point I was changing beds that hadn't even been slept in. And who in their right mind washes clean sheets? So our bed gets changed once (or twice – it depends on the number of wee/poo/unidentifiable spots) a week, and the rest get changed every other week. Ish.

9. Potty training is pointless.

Because you don't need to potty train a child who is ready to be potty trained. And you'll save yourself an *awful* lot of washing. I've learnt that the hard way, and it's a mistake I won't be making again.

First time mum me started to potty train at two and finished at three. Second time mum me started potty training at three and finished at four. Third time mum me didn't need to do anything at all because she just copied the others, so four times mum me won't bother.

Because the thing is you can cajole, encourage, reward, bribe, and beg but you can't make them do their business on the loo. And the sooner you accept that, the better.

The first time around I did it all by the book – literally. We started at two, in the summer - the theory being you can be outside a lot and there's less washing to deal with (there isn't). We had a potty in every room of the house, under the pushchair, and in the back of the car, but still managed to ruin the carpets, the pushchair, and what was once quite a decent car seat. We got there in the end, but arguing with a smaller version of yourself about how to use a toilet *isn't* what I thought motherhood would be about.

So we left it until three the next time, the theory being it wouldn't be as much of an ordeal and there'd be less washing to deal with (it was and there still isn't). Max was four by the time he finally 'got it', which was *so* much older than his peers and I was tearing my hair out dealing with code browns. He simply wasn't interested and was quite happy to walk around in his own sh*t. He'd get taken into the toddler unit at nursery to have his nappy changed because they didn't have a nappy changing unit in the preschool department, but even that wasn't enough to shame him into sitting on the throne.

He was quite happy in nappies, so I gave up. Although changing nappies is a pain in the bum, so is potty training a child who isn't ready. And I've never heard of a teenager who isn't toilet trained. Then, with starting school looming, the unthinkable happened: he just woke up one day, sat on the loo and that was that. No potty training required. He went from nappies to pants in the space of a day, and I can count on one hand the number of accidents he had.

An added bonus was that Marigold (then two) had been watching my vain attempts to get her brother to use the loo, and when he finally did she copied him. So there was no need to potty train her at all. We didn't even need a potty.

As a result, I won't be potty training our lockdown baby. It's too much faff, and totally unnecessary because I've learnt the hard way you don't need to potty train a child who is ready to be potty trained. Plus the older they are the quicker they'll learn to wipe their own bum. And let's face it, there's enough wiping when it comes to parenthood as it is. Why make work for yourself?

10. Lockdown laundry was a blessing in disguise.

There was no school uniform to wash, no 'presents' from nursery in neatly tied up nappy sacks to die at the bottom of the dirty laundry basket (or on top of the washing mountain), and no clothes to worry about not ironing.

We still had a washing mountain and we still needed to call Stuart to come and take it away, but as lockdown went on it became more of a hill than a mountain (the inconceivable happened: the curve flattened itself!) and calls to Stuart became fewer and far between. Then with the help of a heatwave, the kids spent most of the summer naked, or in just pants at best. When it came to washing lockdown and a heatwave was the perfect combination.

You'd *think* a global pandemic would mean you'd need to do more washing, not less, but even with the arrival of Violet at the start of the first lockdown for the first time in years, our washing mountain became almost manageable. Almost.

I no longer needed to go through the washing mountain looking for holes or defects for an excuse to throw things away, and I didn't need to worry about people *seeing* the washing mountain and judging me for it either, because there was no one to see it. Except for the postman (our open bedroom door is next to the front door), but as we've already established in confessions from the lady with the boobs, he's seen *far worse*. The washing mountain is probably the least worse thing he could see (assuming I've remembered to remove the skid-marked inside-out pants stuck inside inside-out trousers, that is).

Of course, the washing mountain is now back to pre-pandemic levels and no doubt it will make me do more funny things, but the bigger it gets the less I care. Because if there's one thing that parenting in a pandemic has taught me it's that keeping everyone alive without killing each other is what matters. Dirty pants, socks, and skid-marked inside-out pants, not so much.

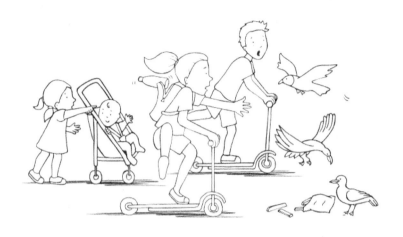

Chapter 8:
Turning into *that* family

Confessions of a mama determined to have a nice time: chasing dough balls, the truth about salt and pepper on restaurant tables, and why it's best just to stay home and stay safe.

THAT family. You know the ones I mean: the ones you can hear coming before you can see them. The ones who cause *some* sort of disturbance as soon as they enter a room. The ones who rearrange restaurant tables and chairs before they've even sat down. The ones you *swore* you'd never become.

There's no getting away from it: as a family of six we are now officially THAT family. Looking back I'd say we started turning into THAT family shortly after the arrival of baby number three. It was being outnumbered by little people that did it. Tell-tale signs you're turning into THAT family include diners on tables nearest to you paying up and leaving within 10 minutes of your arrival at a restaurant. It's *possible* they had actually finished their meals and were about to leave anyway, but the chances are they want to get as far away from you as possible. As fast as possible.

Some sort of spillage will also be involved. And I don't mean a little splash – I mean the sort of spillage that requires reams and reams of the kitchen's catering-size blue roll. The kids will also take it upon themselves to display feral behaviour you've *honestly* never seen before. Like chasing a discarded dough ball around a restaurant floor and then fighting over it. Even though they know we're in the middle of a global pandemic and the five-second rule no longer exists.

So, after four babies - including an accidental lockdown one - here's what I wish I'd known about turning into THAT family:

1. Turning into THAT family is inevitable when you're outnumbered.

It's not a case of if, it's a case of when. And the sooner you accept it and make the best of it, the better. It's a simple case of maths: there's two of you (or one if you're insane enough to go out without backup) and in our case four of them, so *of course* you're going to turn into THAT family at some point.

Realities you need to accept include needing tables with plenty of extra space in restaurants, and if there isn't one you have to rearrange the furniture so that there is. Because not only have you brought the pushchair *and* the car seat with you on the off chance they fall asleep even though everyone knows they won't, the highchair also has to be *at least* a foot away from the edge of the table so the baby is out of swiping distance.

The kids will also probably say something they shouldn't. VERY loudly. Like 'Daddy are you *sure* you can drive us home when you've had two glasses of beer?' And despite using almost a whole pack of baby wipes to clear up all the discarded food, despite putting all the crayons back in their pot, and despite helping to stack the dirty plates, your table *still* looks like a bomb's hit it. Then you leave an overly generous tip. Not because the service was anything special, but in recognition of the trail of destruction you've left in your wake and the general inconvenience caused to all.

The chances are you'll also leave the restaurant with a child under your arm (or one under each arm if it's been an especially bad outing). Because if you haven't marched out of a room carrying a kicking and screaming child under one arm are you even a parent?

2. You open your mouth and your mum falls out.

And not in a good way. You find yourself saying things like 'turn the volume down' and 'other people are here to have a quiet meal and don't want to hear your voice' when what you really mean is that *you* don't want to hear their voice. And you inwardly cringe, but you just can't help yourself.

Just like turning into THAT family, I find myself saying and doing things that my mum said and did when I was young that I *swore* I'd never do. Like saying 'play nicely' and making homemade popcorn to take to the cinema because I can't bring myself to shell out for the over-the-counter stuff. I've also fallen into the trap of saying things like 'we'll see', even though everyone knows that 'we'll see' almost always means no. And 'I'm not going to ask you again', even though everyone knows full well you will. And 'there are children in the world who don't have anything', which, sadly, is still the case.

Once you start turning the music down on the car radio to see better there's no going back. (A post-pandemic equivalent is taking your mask down to hear better, which I've actually found myself doing. I'm guessing it's a slippery slope from now on). If I ever say 'simmer down' or 'wind your neck in' or start cleaning their faces with a licked tissue someone please shoot me.

3. Backwards maths becomes second nature.

And you need backwards maths every time you leave the house. If you haven't had the pleasure yet backwards maths involves establishing what time you need to be somewhere, then working backwards in 30-minute increments factoring in all the things that need to happen in order to actually get out of the door. Then when you've got that figure in your head, which is typically around two hours before you need to be wherever it is you're going, add on 30 minutes 'buffer time' to deal with things you can't plan for. Like the poonami that requires a full-on bath and the cereal that ends up all over the kitchen floor because you stupidly decided to let them pour it themselves. You never know quite what it is that's going to require buffer time, but you can guarantee there'll be something.

4. Back to school shopping with a licky five-year-old and a newborn in a pandemic is a BAD idea.

Especially if you decide to do it on a bank holiday. On your own. By bus. In hindsight, I don't know *what* possessed me. Bluebell later described it as hell on earth, and she wasn't wrong. Lockdown doolallyness must have really got to me because for *some* reason I can't fathom I thought it would be a good idea to take all four kids back to school shopping on August bank holiday Monday. Restrictions were easing, shops and restaurants were opening up again and the ghost buses that had been going past our house totally empty for months were filling up with eager faces.

What I *hadn't* taken into account and had completely forgotten is that I hadn't actually been out on my own with all four kids yet. And that Max was a licky five-year-old with absolutely *no* concept of a link between his tongue, germs, and a global pandemic.

It all started at the bus stop when I realised I'd never taken the pram on a bus before and the front wheels had a mind of their own. There's nothing like a bus load of total strangers staring at you while the driver drums his fingers impatiently on the steering wheel as you try to manoeuvre a buggy that doesn't want to be manoeuvred into position to bring you out in a sweat. Max and Marigold then spent the entire journey trying to touch – and on one occasion lick - the stop bell buttons, and I spent the entire journey telling them not to, sanitising their hands and wondering if I could sanitise their tongues too.

Then when we got into town and the bus spat us out (because that's how it felt) Max took it upon himself to lick a giant ice cream. I don't mean a real ice cream. I mean a plastic one the same height as he was designed to advertise the selling of ice cream that had seen far better days. He put his arms around it, dry-humped it, got as close as he possibly could to it, and ran his tongue all over it. You couldn't make it up. I can laugh about it now, but at the time it was terrible.

The trip continued to go downhill from there. Highlights (or lowlights depending on which way you look at it) included Marigold needing a wee but of course all the toilets were closed; Violet needing a feed but of course the shopping centre nursing room was shut, and forgetting to take socks for the dreaded back to school shoe shopping which despite pre-bookable shoe fitting appointments and social distancing in place of the usual first come first served ticketing system was still a bun fight and *total* chaos.

The final straw came in Marks and Spencer when I turned around and Max was spreadeagled face down on the floor, swishing his arms and legs about like the angel he wasn't because he said it 'felt nice'. Of course Marigold copied him, at which point I did what we should have done in the first place: I herded them into the lift, retreated to the safety of the M&S café, hid in a booth, and called Misery Guts to come and pick us up. Suffice to say we won't be doing *that* again.

5. Eating out to help out didn't help.

Or it didn't help *us* out, anyway. It just served to remind me why I'd rather starve than eat with my kids (see weaning and confessions from the splash mat for the full explanation). As the nation made the most of half-price dinners and dining out for the first time in months with the Eat Out to Help Out scheme, the incentive simply confirmed what I already knew but hoped *might* have changed since the last time we attempted to eat out as a family: my kids will happily chase a discarded dough ball around a restaurant floor and when they've caught it, fight over it. Even though they can't possibly be hungry, know full well we're *still* in the middle of a global pandemic and that the five-second rule will never exist ever again.

That said, there were some silver linings to eating out with the kids. Social distancing and the two-metre rule meant that we no longer needed to rearrange restaurant tables and chairs before we'd even sat down because they'd already been rearranged. There was room for the pushchair *and* the car seat you'd brought with you on the off chance they fall asleep even though everyone knows they won't *and* the highchair that needs to be at least a foot away from the edge of the table so the baby is out of swiping distance.

Diners on tables nearest to us no longer paid up and left within 10 minutes of our arrival in order to get as far away from us as possible, partly because they were as grateful as we were to be 'out out' even if it did mean being sat next to THAT family, but mostly because we were already suitably - and pleasingly - distanced.

There were one or two downsides though. There were no cups of sweaty crayons to entertain the kids in lieu of the ones you could have sworn were in the nappy bag but aren't, and you couldn't let them run off the ice cream sundaes you bought them as a bribe for sitting still while you ate your meal either, because everyone had to stay sat at their table. Even when the meal cost half the price it usually did you still went home wondering why you'd bothered going out in the first place.

6. Never use salt and pepper left on restaurant tables. Ever.

I don't mean salt and pepper they bring out with your food. I mean salt and pepper mills already on your table when you get there. And *definitely* don't use them if we've been sat at the table before you.

They say menus are the dirtiest items to be found in a restaurant, but when kids are the diners I'm willing to bet there's something worse. And my money's on the salt and pepper mills. Pre-kids me didn't give a second thought to salt and pepper mills on restaurant tables, but veteran mum me clocks them and moves them out of reach before our bums have hit the seats.

Because not only do you have no idea when they were last cleaned (or if that cleaning was, in fact, just a cursory wipe) you have no way of knowing how many times they've been accidentally dipped – or double dipped – in other people's dinners. They also tend to be shiny and made of glass and irresistible to little people. Little people who by definition can have quite disgusting things on their hands and about their person, like dribble and bogeys, and worse. And if they're anything like mine, they might also be a bit licky.

I shudder to think how many snot and saliva-laced condiments pre-kids me unwittingly sprinkled on food. It's probably best not to know. Thankfully a Covid silver lining is an end to salt and pepper on restaurant tables. And sauces like ketchup and mayonnaise, which are breeding grounds for all the same reasons. You don't want to be using those either, *especially* if my family has been there first.

7. Seagulls can attack kids.

Living by the sea you'd *think* I'd know this. You'd think I'd know that a seagull the size of a small dog has no qualms about swooping down on a small child and scaring the wits out of them before adding insult to injury by nicking their chips. But a bit like back to school shopping with a licky five-year-old, lockdown doolallyness must have got to me what with the excitement of being able to go 'out out' again. Leading to an unfortunate incident involving a flock of seagulls and not one, not two but three of the four kids. Made worse by the fact that the reason I wasn't there to defend them was because I was buying wine.

It had all been going swimmingly up until that point, too. With pubs and restaurants closed, I'd hit on the idea of fish and chips on the beach for Father's Day. It was the perfect solution: the kids could run about on the beach until their heart's content, we'd get to enjoy a meal out without feeling like THAT family, and if there was some sort of spillage it wouldn't matter. What could possibly go wrong? Instead, the outing turned into the perfect storm.

We did what you always do and got the kids sorted out and eating first. Happily tucking into fish and chips on the pebbles, cans of pop by their side, Misery Guts queued up a few paces away to get our food and I queued up a few paces the other way to get a couple of glasses of wine. I was watching the kids and thinking what a lovely day we were all having when Marigold decided to stand up and walk away from her chips. And anyone who lives by the seaside (me included) will tell you *never* walk away from the chips.

Within seconds a swarm of seagulls was hovering, and seconds after that they were diving. To give Marigold her due she realised what she'd done and did go back to reclaim her chips, but by then it was too late and the seagulls were diving on her – and Bluebell and Max - too. So she screamed and dropped them, sending chips – and seagulls – flying across the promenade with Misery Guts and I *just* out of reach.

It was one of those situations where you can see what's about to happen but can't do anything about it. I can still see the whole debacle playing out in slow motion in my mind: kids crying, seagulls dive-bombing, and Violet sleeping innocently in her pram in the middle of all the commotion. Hats off to the great British public though, who rushed to their aid as I sprinted towards them, all thoughts of a pandemic and social distancing temporarily forgotten in the face of a more immediate emergency.

So we turned into THAT family again after all, and to add salt to the wound now it's my fault the kids are afraid of seagulls. Which is a bit unfortunate given that we live by the sea.

8. It's surprisingly easy to turn a garden igloo into a dutch oven.

I don't mean a heavy cooking pot with a tight-fitting lid. I mean trapping your nearest and dearest and an unsuspecting waitress in a confined space with a cloud of eye-watering farts. All you need is a trumping child. Or four.

Like banana bread and sourdough starters, garden igloos also had a moment in lockdown when they popped up everywhere from hotels and restaurants to schools and back gardens to get around social distancing rules and the great British weather.

As an outnumbered mum of four with a licky five-year-old and a little sister who copies *everything* he does the garden igloo craze seemed like the perfect solution when it came to going 'out out'. We'd be contained and safely zipped into our own private space, the kids wouldn't be able to chase dough balls under other people's tables, other diners wouldn't be able to hear us and we wouldn't be able to hear *them* tutting or making disapproving comments at the way we weren't bringing up the kids.

So when a local restaurant transformed their garden into an Instagrammable winter wonderland featuring igloos complete with fairy lights, cascading bunches of artificial flowers, sheepskin rugs, and individual heaters to see them through the winter months I'd booked one before you could say the word 'igloo'.

It was early December, it was dark at four o'clock, our igloo was lit up with magical twinkly fairy lights, and inside was warm and cosy with one button to press for table service and another for the heater. We were 'out out' for the first time in months and for the first time as a family of six I wasn't going to feel like THAT family.

But while it was true that we were contained and safely zipped into our own private space, the kids couldn't chase dough balls under other people's tables, other diners couldn't hear us and we couldn't hear them, what I *didn't* appreciate is how being safely zipped into our own private space would play out in reality.

Within minutes one of the kids had let one go. Except owing to the fact we were safely zipped inside a garden igloo there was nowhere *for* it to go, so it hung about in a farty cloud above our heads and under the magical twinkly fairy lights. The parp (eventually) petered out, leaving a lingering sour twang in the air, but by then one of them had let another one go (you can see where this is going). So the whole process started again, only it was slightly worse this time because the second parp was on top of the last one with a second lingering sour twang on top of the last one.

Before we knew it farty condensation was running down the inside of the igloo, fuelled by a surprisingly efficient patio heater, and what can only be described as fart juice was pooling onto the floor. Every time the waitress unzipped our door to bring more drinks we gulped in the fresh air, and she visibly recoiled despite having the benefit and added protection of a face mask. I actually saw her eyes water.

When Violet decided to fill her nappy I knew it was time to go. The fumage was even making *my* eyes water, and I'm used to it. I'm also pretty sure the methane generated by our igloo alone would have been classed as a fire hazard. As we bid a hasty exit I made sure to double-check that none of our fellow diners had stepped outside their igloos for a quick smoke, because they'd have got more than they bargained for.

So, yet again and somewhat inevitably, we turned into THAT family. And, if you'll excuse the pun, it turns out garden igloos aren't all they're cracked up to be.

9. Being determined to have a nice time is a waste of time.

And being determined to have a nice time means you probably won't. Thanks to unforeseen events you simply can't plan for like rogue dough balls, seagull attacks, and dutch ovens. The saying goes best-laid plans go to waste for a reason.

Instead, it's *far* better to lower your expectations to rock bottom, which is a solid foundation from which things can only turn out better than you expected. And actually, it's on those occasions that you end up having the nicest time. The outings you *thought* were going to go horribly wrong owing to things like food you know they won't eat and danger nap time turn out to be the days pre-parent you pictured. At the time of writing, I can't actually think of any (I asked Misery Guts and he can't, either) but I'm pretty sure there must have been some. Or it could be a figment of my sleep-deprived imagination.

10. Sometimes it's best just to stay at home to stay safe.

I don't mean to avoid catching and spreading Covid. I mean to avoid catching and spreading farts in igloos. And dribble and bogeys on salt and pepper mills. And dough balls on restaurant floors. As a family of six when it comes to being out in public *en masse* I've discovered that sometimes (most of the time) it's best just to stay at home to stay safe. Especially in the midst of a global pandemic. (The alternative is to divide and conquer, but we'll get to that in confessions of corona mummy and finding our new normal).

Until such a time that we *don't* need to rearrange restaurant tables and chairs before we've sat down, don't turn garden igloos into dutch ovens, and don't cause some sort of hullabaloo everywhere we go, I've decided it's probably best to avoid falling into THAT family situations altogether. Because it's not possible to be seen and not heard. I can categorically say you will *always* hear us coming before you can see us. Sorry not sorry.

"Writing swear words in alphabites is surprisingly therapeutic"

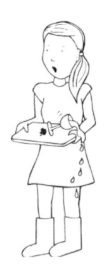

Chapter 9:
The myth of having it all

Confessions of a mama doing too many things and none of them well: why there's nothing wrong with being 'just' a mum, the day I told the Chancellor of the Exchequer to f*ck off in alphabites, and embracing the (puree-splatted) glass ceiling.

They say the secret to having it all is knowing you already do. But that doesn't help much when you've got 157 unread school WhatsApp messages (not to mention 99 unread breakout group WhatsApp messages); an online Big Shop to finalise;

a work deadline looming; a washing mountain with school uniform needed yesterday at the summit and a scale model of an Egyptian pyramid to make by 8 o'clock tomorrow morning.

And funnily enough, the more kids you've got the more plates you've got to spin. Which is blindingly obvious when you think about it. But the trouble is I *didn't* think about it. Not until I suddenly found myself spinning them, and by then it was too late. Four kids is *a lot* of plates. And four kids and a pandemic is even more plates. Something (or someone) has to give – or fall off completely and smash on the floor. As a result, my standards have lowered with each child, and a lot of the time I feel like I'm doing too many things and none of them well.

So, after four babies - including an accidental lockdown one - here's what I wish I'd known about the myth of having it all:

1. You can't have it all.

First time mum me *thought* you could, but you can't. And if you insist on going after it you'll probably die trying. Or go mad. Or both.

Looking back it all started as soon as I had baby number one. I was the news editor of a series of local tabloid newspapers, with five paid-for and three free titles published each week. There were print deadlines on three of my five working days, and the culture was to stay in the office until the paper was put to bed. But the thing is, I wanted to put my baby to bed, not a newspaper.

After becoming a mum I simply couldn't see myself in the role anymore, and I didn't want to fall into the trap of over-compensating for the fact I needed to be out of the office door by six o'clock every day by doing more work than anyone else when I was there and then legging it to pick-up with seconds to spare like so many of us do.

So I took the plunge and went freelance, slowly building a new career and fitting work around nappy changes and talking tots classes. I did the same again with baby number two, taking just nine weeks maternity leave because I was self-employed and that's all we could afford, and by the time I was expecting baby number three I was working full time hours around two little people and a (rather large) bump. But like pumping milk at work, it turns out that was unsustainable too.

By the time Marigold arrived and I went back to work after maternity leave there was no way I could work full-time hours and look after three little people during the day at the same time, so I did what I could. There were (and still are) work opportunities I simply couldn't go after anymore owing to childcare duties and the unpaid work needed to be done at home.

While Misery Guts' career as a magazine editor went from strength to strength, my career went in the opposite direction. It stopped and started because of maternity leave, and then, when back working again, I desperately grappled with deadlines between school and nursery runs, ferrying children to and from clubs and doing all the things you need to do with them while he was at work.

Then the pandemic struck and we all know what happened then. Lockdown served to make the inequalities worse because I finished work to go on maternity leave the day they closed down the country, so somewhat inevitably (and very grudgingly) it fell to me to look after the kids so Misery Guts could work full time and pay the bills. By the time we emerged from Lockdown 3 and almost without noticing we'd slowly but surely slipped into traditional nuclear family roles, with Misery Guts the breadwinner and me looking after the kids. And I hate it. I hate the fact that it's childcare arrangements that allow me to work.

The trouble is society wants you to *think* you can have it all, which is how I found myself pumping breastmilk on a closed toilet seat while desperately chasing my dream job after baby number two (see breastfeeding and confessions from the lady with the boobs if you're not already familiar with the sorry tale). But I realised very quickly after returning to work that it was breastfeeding or the job – I couldn't have both.

Social media doesn't help either, with pop stars and Olympians and models filling their squares with snapshots of them going about their hugely successful careers with a baby strapped to their chest or a breast pump (or two) attached to a boob. But as we all know it takes a village to raise a child, and those pop stars and Olympians and models not only have a village but no money worries and an invisible city beavering away behind their grids, without whom none of it would be possible.

But of course, you don't see that when you're sat at home scrolling on your phone in your leggings with your mum bun in a house that looks like a bomb's hit it. You see a pop star or an Olympian or a model living their best life, and you wonder where you went wrong. Except you didn't go wrong. You had kids. And the chances are they probably haven't got it all and they're probably not living their best lives, either.

There's also nothing wrong with *wanting* to have it all even though you know you can't. Because you're still a human with hopes and dreams, even if it doesn't feel like it sometimes. Plus it's human nature to want what you can't have.

2. There's nothing wrong with being 'just' a mum.

Being 'just' a mum is often considered a demeaning term, the implication being that being a mum is less important or valuable than, for example, a nurse or a scientist. You never hear anyone say I'm 'just a nurse' or I'm 'just a scientist'. But I don't see it in a derogatory sense at all. *Of course* there's so much more to all of us than motherhood, but the truth is being 'just' a mum can also be a relief.

As a stay-and-work-at-home mum I feel like I'm constantly being pulled in two completely opposite – and impossible – directions. In the run-up to all my maternity leaves I couldn't *wait* to be 'just' a mum. I couldn't wait to be doing just one job – mumming – instead of mumming *and* trying to earn money at the same time.

Of course, being a mum is a far cry from just one job – you're an alarm clock, a cook, a cleaner, a wiper upper, a housekeeper, a Big Shop booker, a children's entertainer, an account manager, and the list goes on – but when you're trying to earn money as well there comes a point when the juggling gets in the way of the joy. If you take away some of that juggling you can replace it with the joy again, which makes being 'just' a mum fine by me.

3. All mums are working mums.

And while we're on the subject of labels, all mums are full-time mums too. Because you don't stop being a mum the moment you sit down at a computer and walk into an office. It doesn't matter whether you're a high-flying city banker mum, a teacher mum, a work-from-home mum, or a stay-at-home mum, you're still a working mum.

Just because you don't get paid for it doesn't make the job any less valid or important. In fact, I'd go as far as to say being a stay-at-home mum is harder than any job with a salary, because you're wearing so many different hats at the same time, and many of the tasks required are not only menial but mind-numbingly repetitive and boring. You also don't get the perks that come with a salaried job, like lunch, tea, and coffee breaks, weeing in peace, annual leave, and a pension. And there's no one to go out for drinks with afterwards, either. (Although on the flip side, there's also no one to tell you off for drinking on the job, as we've already established in homeschooling hell and confessions of a (very) reluctant teacher).

4. Being a stay-and-work-at-home mum isn't the best of both worlds.

It sounds like the dream scenario: working flexibly around the kids, being there for all the milestones, reading bedtime stories, and being the one to wipe away the tears. If it wasn't for the fact a lot of the tears you end up wiping are your own.

I thought being a stay-and-work-at-home mum would be the answer to all my mum guilt problems: I could exclusively breastfeed, I'd be there for all the 'firsts', I could even do it in my jim jams if necessary while still contributing to the family finances and retaining some sense of my former self. And while working from home did indeed allow me to do all those things, it's also the toughest job I've ever had.

On a bad day it's astonishing just how little it's possible to achieve. From the empty breakfast bowls and soggy cornflakes you need to chisel off the table before you can start work to the beds that haven't been made yet and the dishwasher that hasn't been emptied, it can feel like you've already done a day's work before you've even started your own (paid) work.

Then there's the fact that being at home all day means the house gets messy in a way it just wouldn't if everyone was out at work, school and nursery. It gets dusty quicker, needs hoovering more often, the bins fill up in the blink of an eye and before you know it you're back to cleaning up again (you can see the cycle that's emerging here).

Then there's the dreaded call from school or nursery to come and pick them up because they've puked, coughed, or are running a slight temperature. You're the one at home so it falls to you to do the collecting and the cuddling, and although you're there to make it all better, inside your heart is sinking because you know you're going to have to work in the evening and possibly at the weekend to make up for it.

And it's not just lifemin and little people who disrupt your day. Grown-ups do too, and they should know better. It never ceases to amaze me the assumptions people make when you work from home, like thinking they can 'pop in' for a cup of tea when they wouldn't dream of 'popping in' to an office, hospital, or shop uninvited in the middle of the working day. Then there are the people who ask you do to things like help with cake sales or pick something up for them 'seeing as you work from home' and take offence when you say you can't because you're working. They're also the ones most likely to ask why you send the children to nursery when you work from home, and the ones I'm most likely to want to punch in the face. With a little bit of luck after lockdown there'll be fewer of those about now.

I used to envy Misery Guts his 45-minute drive to and from work when he could sit alone in peace without anyone wanting or needing anything or shouting *muuum* ten million times. He couldn't understand it – until he went freelance himself. Now he *totally* gets it (along with why, at the end of the day, there was a *huge* difference between him leaving the office on time or half an hour later). Now he works from home too I know he goes outside to do the bins just to get away from it all, and I'm pretty sure he sits in the car just to get a bit of peace and quiet too. So you see, being a stay-and-work-at-home mum (or dad) isn't actually a dream scenario at all. On a bad day it can be more like a nightmare.

5. Never underestimate the power of a crisp sandwich.

Or a nipple. Or a smartie. (Not for you, for them – although to be fair it doesn't get much better than a crisp sandwich for lunch when you work from home). Over the years things I've used to occupy and keep the kids quiet while working from home include my nipples (not both at the same time, obviously) smarties, and crisps sandwiches. Nipples for the milk when I was breastfeeding, smarties because the tiniest snack possible takes them the longest possible time to eat, which is just the job for phone and conference calls, and crisp sandwiches for the same reason.

Letting them make things like their own crisp sandwiches may *sound* like a false economy owing to the mess you'll be clearing up later, but it'll buy you the time you need in the short term and you'll be surprised how long it takes them to carry out the *simplest* task. A crisp sandwich, for example, will generally free up a good 20 minutes. Admittedly the butter looks like it's been attacked with a machete afterwards but in the short term think of the 20 minutes.

The TV is also your friend, and forget what they say about screen time - they're *not* going to get square eyes from staring at a screen. And so what if the baby knows which button to press when the notification on the telly pops up telling you it's been on so long it's about to switch off. That's actually quite clever.

6. The motherhood penalty is alive and kicking.

In fact, it's everywhere you look, only I didn't notice until I became a mum. And the more kids you've got, the greater that penalty is. It all starts when maternity leave takes you (temporarily) out of the office and everyone else carries on with their career and you don't. Then once you're back in the game and can swap mumwear for workwear again you probably need them to be a bit flexible to fit around drop-offs and pick-ups and sick days, but they don't like that. Then a few years after that you discover that school holidays and annual leave don't add up, and you don't have to understand improper fractions to know there's absolutely *no way* four weeks annual leave (or five if you're lucky) is going to cover 13 weeks of school holidays.

They say having a baby is expensive, but what I didn't appreciate is the cost of having a baby (or four) to my career. After four pregnancies (six actually, but we'll come to that in confessions of an accidental mum of four), four maternity leaves, and 10 years of motherhood I now feel so far behind that I'll never be able to catch up.

And that motherhood penalty continues. The pandemic is a prime example, when the government introduced the Self-Employment Income Support Scheme to help self-employed people like me whose incomes were affected by the crisis. Payments were calculated based on profits in previous tax years, but if you happened to have been on maternity leave during those tax years the amount you were entitled to was affected, because you were considered not working and 'economically inactive'.

But the thing is, I wasn't not working and I wasn't economically inactive either. Maternity leave isn't a holiday. I simply wasn't doing *paid* work. I was doing unpaid work raising a future doctor or nurse or vaccine inventor or prime minister. But they don't care about that, because on paper you're 'just' a mum.

7. Writing swear words in alphabites is surprisingly therapeutic.

Especially when you're telling the Chancellor of the Exchequer to f*ck off with them. There were two things that drove me to it: the powers that be releasing a new 'stay home, save lives' poster, which featured illustrations of women cooking, cleaning, and homeschooling while a man did nothing but sit on a sofa, and the Chancellor of the Exchequer having the audacity to 'thank mums' for juggling homeschooling with everything else during Lockdown 3.

The poster was very quickly withdrawn by the Government, and the Chancellor of the Exchequer was very quickly called out by a consternation of inner rage-fuelled mums, but it was too late and the damage was done. The fact that the people running the country thought it was ok to perpetuate the idea that childcare, household duties, and homeschooling are 'women's work' made (and still makes) me *so* angry. What's equally alarming is that that poster would have been briefed, commissioned, designed, finalised, and gone through numerous rounds of proofing before it made it to print, yet *no one* thought to point out it depicted women doing *all* the things and one man doing absolutely nothing. I was so cross I even shouted at Alexa that day, and she's usually my sidekick.

I was angrily throwing frozen food onto a baking tray and lamenting the unfairness of it all when I realised what it was that would make me feel better. Telling the Chancellor of the Exchequer to f*ck off in alphabites. The trouble is I couldn't actually write f*ck off, because

I didn't have enough vowels. I didn't have enough fs either, but as an editor once said to me never let the truth get in the way of a good story. I fashioned the letters I needed by biting bits off other consonants, which also made me feel better. (In hindsight I should have turned the activity into a homeschooling lesson, although I'm not quite sure what the subject would be. I don't think it could technically be classed as home economics). Either way, the episode temporarily diffused my anger and we all laughed for the first time in ages. Even Misery Guts.

Other therapeutic uses for alphabites include writing rude words you know they can't read with them, and propositioning each other because you know if you put the tea in they'll go and check on it and discover your naughty message when they slide out the baking tray. Until one day you discover the kids can suddenly read them and you find yourself having to explain what a minge is.

8. Embracing the (puree-splatted) glass ceiling is REALLY liberating.

A bit like the realisation there's absolutely nothing wrong with being 'just' a mum, accepting there's a (puree-splatted) glass ceiling is actually really liberating.

I'm not saying it's right and I'm not saying we shouldn't all be doing what we can to challenge - and change – the motherhood penalty and the status quo, I'm saying there's a lot to be said for accepting the situation for what it is. For example, I spent my twenties establishing and building a career. In my thirties I was then in a position to be able to take a step back and focus on starting a family while going freelance and (just about) keep the money coming in. Then in my forties, with childbearing and breastfeeding (almost) out of the way, I hope to be able to focus on my career again.

I'm not saying it's right to be forced to choose between motherhood and a career and then to find yourself winging it doing both, but by accepting there's a (puree-splatted) glass ceiling and doing things like writing swear words in alphabites you won't be so perma-cross.

9. It's not easier to do it all yourself than ask for help.

First time mum me *thought* it was easier to do it all myself rather than ask for help, mainly because I tend to be over-prepared and other people tend to be under-f*cking prepared (the flashing fuel light in confessions from the head end is a perfect example). And if someone does something and it's not the way I do it, like folding towels, I'll do it again.

But four times mum me knows it *isn't* easier to do it all yourself than ask for help. Because you can't do everything, and if you try you'll burn out eventually. You simply can't do *all the things* all the time. I know because I've been there, done it, spun the plates, and picked up the broken ones that have crashed to the floor. (I'll still re-fold the towels if you've done them wrong though).

10. Pandemic parenting *might* have been a good thing.

Bear with me on this one. As horrendous, thankless, invisible, exhausting, stressful, and traumatic as pandemic parenting was, there *is* a chance something good might come out of it. Because the crisis shone a light on another kind of crisis that's been going on for years: the motherhood penalty and the ongoing and relentless daily paid-unpaid work juggle. I'm willing to bet that post-pandemic fewer people will ask what it is stay-at-home parents actually *do* all day.

Until the pandemic we were expected to work as if we don't have children, and raise children as if we don't work. The pandemic exposed that uncomfortable truth, and something good might come out of that. I don't know quite *what* yet, but something might.

"You can make lists and add things to calendars and still have absolutely no idea what's going on"

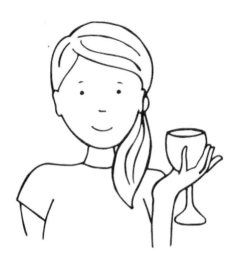

Chapter 10:

Mental load

Confessions of a mama at the end of her rope: the day a DJ saved my life, track and tracing the old me, and locking down a mum-life balance.

One hundred and seventy three. That's how many times the kids said, shouted, or screamed '*muuum*' (or a variation of it) in just one hour during a particularly testing day in lockdown. And every day was testing. I know because I counted, just to prove to Misery Guts that it would be more than one hundred. And there's only so many times you can hear the word 'muuum' (or a variation of it) until you either want to scream too or hide in a dark cupboard where there's no hope of them finding you. Which is a bit difficult when you live in a two-bedroom flat with four kids.

Lockdown aside though, another thing first time mum me didn't appreciate is the mental load and the invisible, intangible work that comes with parenthood. Like booking online Big Shops, RSVP'ing to party invites, paying after school club invoices, and knowing when a plastic bottle with the top cut off is needed for Brownies. And the more of you there are, the more there is to remember, organise, account for, plan, and manage. Sometimes it feels like my head could explode with things that aren't written down anywhere but need to be done. And if I don't do them, they won't happen.

So, after four babies - including an accidental lockdown one - here's what I wish I'd known about mental load:

1. Bad days don't make bad mums.

Even if the day in question is *really* bad, bad days don't make bad mums. You're simply a good mum having a bad day. As a mama of four there have been *lots* of bad days over the years, ranging from accidentally weeing on the arms of jumpsuits in confessions from the lady with the boobs (not my proudest moment) to the hoover and the haddock incident in weaning and confessions from the splash mat. But the worst days were without doubt during lockdown when life became a pressure cooker of juggling maternity leave and then work with looking after the kids, homeschooling, and all the unseen jobs that come with family life.

Because of the pandemic some of those invisible, intangible tasks which had previously been annoying but pretty straightforward were also suddenly impossible, like booking the online Big Shop. Within days of the first lockdown supermarket home delivery slots were rarer than hen's teeth and getting one felt like winning the jackpot – a mental load kind of jackpot, but a jackpot nonetheless. Each week, still recovering from giving birth and eyes stinging with tiredness, I'd stay up until way past midnight refreshing the supermarket webpage just to bag a slot because pandemic or no pandemic, hiding behind a mouse and clicking is *far* preferable than going food shopping with kids.

Luckily my knack of getting my hands on 90s boy band tickets came in rather handy (refreshing a web page is the modern-day equivalent of hitting the redial button on a phone in a split second) and we managed to bag a home delivery slot every week in lockdown. And while it did indeed feel like winning the jackpot, the late-night task also added to an already rather hefty mental load.

It was after the delivery of one of the aforementioned online Big Shops when the driver wasn't allowed into our building to deliver it to our fourth-floor flat owing to new Covid rules, so I had to go down and load it all into the pram and take it up in the lift around a sleeping Violet, that I realised bad days don't make bad mums. Bluebell and I had been grappling with improper fractions (again) when the delivery arrived, and we were both on the verge of tears (again). The arrival of the Big Shop was a welcome diversion, so when we'd ferried the super noodles nobody really likes but I was still buying because it seemed like a sensible thing to do up to the flat and put it all away we called it quits and went to the park instead. Where I had an epiphany, and a DJ saved my life.

Because Fatboy Slim, or Norman Cook to call him by his real name, owns the café at the park closest to our flat. And because of the pandemic he couldn't do his normal day job of DJing, because there was nowhere to DJ, so he swapped his headphones and decks for serving fish finger sandwiches and wine in pint glasses instead. And just like me trying to teach Bluebell how to do improper fractions, to start with he wasn't very good at it. Not the fish finger sandwiches and wine in pint glasses (that was an *excellent* idea and one I took full advantage of) but the taking of orders and the giving of change.

I was watching him struggle with the till as I patiently waited in the queue when it dawned on me: messing up orders and giving the incorrect change didn't make him a bad DJ. He was a DJ getting to grips with something new. And messing up homeschooling and not being able to teach improper fractions didn't make me a bad mum. It made me a mum getting to grips with something new. And that little epiphany cheered me up immensely. So I ordered a fish finger sandwich and a pint of wine, stopped beating myself up about homeschooling (or lack of it) and we didn't cry about improper fractions again.

2. You can't be expected to remember everything.

Like your children's names, for example. Calling the child you want to speak to the first few syllables of the name of everyone else in the house, including the cats, before eventually arriving at the correct name is perfectly normal. Reassuringly normal, in fact.

Even if it is yet another sign you're turning into your mother. Because you can't be expected to remember everything. Not when there's online Big Shops to book, meals to plan, cleaning to do, plastic bottles to remember to cut the tops off, lunches to make, and kids to keep alive.

You also don't want to be adding to the mental load. I vividly recall a conversation with my mum when I was working from home when Max was a baby and doing the two-mile school run on foot because we only had one car and Misery Guts used it for work during the week. She questioned why I bought ready-made bags of snacking cheese at a vastly inflated price for him to eat in the pushchair on the way, instead of cutting up cubes from a block of cheese and putting them in a sandwich bag at a fraction of the price. But it was nothing to do with the price. Or laziness. Cutting up cubes from a block of cheese and bagging them up would have been yet another thing to add to the invisible mental load list inside my head and set aside time for – time I didn't have and a mental load list that was already as long as my arm. The truth is I couldn't put a price on being able to grab a ready-made bag of cheese from the fridge on our way out of the door without having to think about it. The convenience was priceless.

3. RSVP rage is real.

I thought accidentally forgetting to RSVP to kids' party invites owing to mental (over) load wasn't really all that bad. And that RSVP'ing the day before the party late was better than not RSVP'ing at all. But it is and it's not. RSVP rage is real. I know because I've been on the receiving end, all because I didn't go through school and nursery bags sheaf of paper by sheaf of paper and discover the invitation in question at pick up while doing a million other things and being chatted total rubbish at (by the kids I mean, not the host of the party).

The only thing worse than discovering a kids' party invite languishing – unopened – at the bottom of a book bag after the event is receiving a follow-up invitation to one you haven't RSVP'd to yet. Twice I've received handwritten notes from super organised mums politely asking if I've received their invitation and could I please reply, and on both occasions, I've felt absolutely terrible.

But in defence of mamas doing too many things and none of them well RSVP'ing isn't necessarily as straightforward as it sounds. It's not a simple case of spending a few minutes sending a message or a text either way. It's whatever else is going on during those minutes, and the mental load that comes with those minutes.

For example, if you don't already know the parent in question you've got to manually tap their number into your phone, which is easier said than done if you're trying to do it with your non-dominant hand while breastfeeding a baby and cooking tea at the same time. Then you've got to write it on the calendar, which again is easier said than done if you're trying to do it with your non-dominant hand while breastfeeding a baby and cooking tea at the same time.

It's at that point that you decide to make a mental note to do it when things are a bit quieter and a bit less hectic, except they're never a bit quieter and a bit less hectic. Making mental notes to add to the mental load already in your head is a *really* bad idea because they'll almost certainly never happen. And even if you do manage to tap out your RSVP, it's easy to be called away to referee or deal with some child-related emergency before you've hit send and then forget all about it for a week or two, or RSVP and *think* you've hit send without realising until a week or so later that you actually didn't.

I don't mean to do it, yet there always seems to be an RSVP that slips through the net. So the moral of the story is this: go through school and nursery bags sheaf of paper by sheaf of paper and discover the invitation at pick up even if you're doing a million other things while being chatted total rubbish at, RSVP immediately, write it on the calendar even if it means doing it with your non-dominant hand while breastfeeding and cooking tea and whatever happens, remember to actually look at the calendar so you don't forget the big day.

4. Lists don't necessarily make you more organised.

Because you can make lists and add things to calendars and still have absolutely no idea what's going on. Even if you've got lists for your lists. They can *help* you feel more organised, but in practice if all you're doing is transferring the overwhelm from your head to a piece of paper and then constantly adding to it you're no better off than you were before you started the list. All you're really doing is adding to the mental load with another task to work through. Which is a shame because I used to love a list. Instead, I now email myself to remind myself to do things and flag them up as important with a red exclamation mark. The only trouble is there are currently 15, 017 unread messages in my inbox, and most of them have red exclamation marks.

5. It's best not to overthink things.

Otherwise you find yourself having dark thoughts. Like CBeebies dark thoughts, which are especially bad at six o'clock on a Sunday morning when you're a bit hungover and they've been awake since five. These dark thoughts include WTAF the Teletubbies' tubby custard is, whether The Clangers are cannibals because they're made from wool and knit with wool too, and why Teal from The Adventures of Abney & Teal doesn't have rickets owing to the fact he lives on an island and only eats porridge.

It's also best not to overthink things like who invented armpit fudge, how, and why. I'd never come across armpit fudge before until it appeared in the subject line of a Zoom invitation towards the end of Lockdown 3, not long after the condom and the Beaver incident (see homeschooling hell and confessions of a (very) reluctant teacher).

It transpires armpit fudge is exactly that: fudge made with your armpit. Any armpit will do. You simply put all the ingredients in a resealable freezer bag, seal it (it turns out that bit's quite important) then you mix it all together with the power of your armpit until it resembles fudge. The kids found it hysterical and admittedly it *was* quite funny, especially when they started armpit farting too. What wasn't so funny was when it came to making the second batch, and Max forgot the vital second stage: to seal the resealable freezer bag. Let's just say that, like all the cooking activities conducted over Zoom in lockdown, the kitchen floor ended up stickier than a soft play café.

6. Sensory overload doesn't just affect babies.

It affects mamas too. Especially when it comes to being touched out. Why don't they warn you about the touching? I don't mean a slobbery kiss here and a heart-melting hug there, I mean a toddler intent on burrowing their finger as deep as it'll possibly go into your belly button with one hand while fingering all your moles with the other while you feed their baby sister at the same time.

Signs you're touched out include leaping off the sofa if your other half happens to brush your shoulder, either accidentally or on purpose, rolling yourself in the duvet at bedtime so no one can touch you, and locking yourself in the loo just to have a moment to yourself. And it's not surprising when you think about it. You've grown a baby inside your body, fed a baby with your body and then that baby climbs all over you and tramples on your toes every day for the next five years.

Apparently, belly button fiddling and toe trampling are totally normal, but while I sometimes question my own parenting skills, I also question my own kids' kidding skills too.

7. You have to let off steam.

Because if you didn't you'd spontaneously combust. Biting the head off Freddo frogs with your head in a kitchen cupboard is good, as is kicking my way through all the discarded shoes and coats left abandoned on the hall floor and ramming the pushchair wheels over them to get out of the door. *That's* a really good way to let off some steam.

8. A chronic illness doesn't just affect the person who has it.

It affects the whole family - and it has a *big* impact on mental load. I promised to introduce you to Misery Guts properly in chapter one and confessions from the head end and I'm not quite sure why it's taken me until chapter 10 and mental load to do it, but better late than never. Which is what he always is anyway, so this is my chance to get him back.

The truth is Misery Guts is called Misery Guts for good reason. It's because a lot of the time his blood is boiling.

Which makes him angry. And grumpy. And miserable. Not because we're outnumbered or because one of the kids is doing something they shouldn't (although those things too), but because he's got type 1 diabetes and when his blood sugar level is running high his blood really is boiling.

He was diagnosed with type 1 diabetes when he was 12. This means his pancreas doesn't produce any insulin, which helps turn food into energy, so he has to inject it instead. At first he did this via a syringe several times a day, which involved checking his blood sugar level first with another needle. Now he has a pump on his arm to deliver the insulin and a sensor on his other arm to measure his blood sugar level, which we joke makes him part man, part robot. There is currently no cure for type 1 diabetes, meaning all you can do is manage it. It also means his body can't control his blood sugar level, which can be really dangerous if it drops too low – or goes too high.

If it goes too low he can have a hypoglycaemic attack and start to tremble, shake, and even fit. He can become confused as his body shuts down because he doesn't have enough energy and if he doesn't raise his blood sugar level quickly by eating or drinking something sugary he can lose consciousness. This isn't usually a problem during the day – he checks his blood regularly and can feel the symptoms coming on and react accordingly. The problem is at night when he's asleep and not aware of how he's feeling. We've had some pretty close calls over the years resulting in me having no option but to dial 999.

The first time this really hit home was when I was about six months pregnant with Bluebell and his blood sugar level dropped too low. It was three o'clock in the morning and as his body shook and convulsed I tried to get him in the recovery position as I waited for the ambulance to arrive. At the same time I had to protect my bump from his flailing arms and legs. I had to protect my bump from diabetes, which is something that hadn't occurred to me when I stood at the altar saying my vows and promising to look after him in sickness and in health.

A few months later in the delivery suite at the hospital it was *me* asking Misery Guts if he was alright as I breathed through contractions in the middle of the night because anything out of the normal routine plays havoc with blood sugar levels. There were more snacks in our hospital bag for him than there were for me.

And a few years after that, with four children on the scene, life is a delicate balancing act of juggling his blood sugar level with family life. More often than not, when he's losing his patience with the kids or snapping at them (or me) for something they've said or done, it isn't daddy talking, it's the diabetes. And it's *really* important to me that the kids know this.

In a bid to try and make things a bit easier, instead of sharing the invisible load of parenthood like booking online Big Shops, RSVP'ing to kids' party invites, paying after school club invoices, and knowing when plastic bottles with their tops cut off are needed for Brownies I don't because I know he's got his own invisible load to deal with. Diabetes means constantly checking what your blood sugar level is, constantly adjusting insulin amounts in response, constantly working out the correct level of insulin to give yourself based on what you're eating and your activity levels - and guessing what's right when you're not quite sure what's in the food you're going to be eating.

It means having a hypoglycaemic attack if your blood sugar level drops too low and it means running the risk of doing serious damage to your heart and other vital organs if your blood sugar level runs too high. It means not sleeping alone because if you do have a hypoglycaemic attack there's a risk you might not wake up. Which is a *big* mental load. It's exhausting and I don't blame him for being grumpy about it. My blood would be boiling too.

9. Starting a mummy blog saved my sanity.

You can say what you like about mummy bloggers, the fact is starting a mummy blog saved my sanity. When I became a mum in 2011 I suddenly went from working full-time at the beating heart of a tabloid newsroom to being at home on my own all day with a baby who couldn't talk back. And even though she was my baby and I loved my new job, I found myself with lots to say and nobody to say it to.

So I started telling complete strangers about things like the mysterious case of the hoover and the haddock on the internet, which is when Confessions of a Crummy Mummy was born. When I first came up with the moniker I had *no idea* how true it would turn out to be – and just how necessary my little corner of the internet would be to let off steam with like-minded mums and dads.

Through writing about the highs and lows of parenting, sharing experiences, and inviting comments back you quickly discover you're not the only one wondering if fish fingers twice in one week makes you a bad mum, you're not the only one with a threenager you have to bribe to do virtually anything and you're not the only one at the end of their rope.

Over the years I've met so many people, many of whom I count as true friends even though we've never actually met in real life. As a blogger and a person who reads blogs, you learn about the ins and outs of other people's lives, and you're there to support each other virtually through the ups and downs. Which is quite handy when you find yourself locked down in the middle of a global pandemic.

Over the years I've also managed to turn my blog into a business, although I know some people don't think blogging is a proper job. But if creating a brand, building a platform on which to showcase that brand, growing an audience, attracting household names to pay to reach that audience, and running and managing that platform by being a content creator, editor and photographer isn't a 'proper job' I'd love to know what is. My blog is also the book I didn't know I'd written. And now here it is right here in your hands. But if some people prefer to think of blogging as 'just' an online diary by 'just' a mum, that's fine by me.

10. Locking down a mum-life balance is essential to survival.

It might mean swapping spa days and manicures for hiding in the loo and painting your own nails, but establishing some kind of mum-life balance is essential to survival. Especially in a pandemic.

As a stay-and-work-at-home mum I spend pretty much all my time at home – there's no going to work and leaving everything that's going on at home at home until I return in the evening, and there's no coming home and leaving everything that's going on at work at work until I return the following day. Basically, there is *no* escape. So I created one. In the form of an allotment.

It's about the size of the corner of a football pitch, it's got a she-shed I painted bluebell blue on it and I pay the council about £40 a year for the pleasure. I hot-foot it there for a couple of hours child-free at the weekend and if I'm lucky I make it there on summer evenings too. No matter what mood I'm in when I go I always feel better afterwards, and no matter how worn down I'm feeling with the kids just a couple of hours break gives me time to miss them and feel raring to go again. Basically, the break makes me a better mum. Even when I'm not there I'm thinking about it – it's what helps get me through the week. That and wine.

It's also good to have something 'else'. When I say 'else' I mean something that doesn't involve being a mum and something that doesn't involve work either. One of the things I love about it is that I can keep everything in orderly rows and neat and tidy in a way that just isn't possible at home. The allotment is the only place I find just as I left it, give or take a few weeds.

Track and tracing the old you is also essential to survival. Which is how I came to find myself with a personal trainer. At first, it was due to lockdown, when all the gyms and swimming pools were closed and I couldn't run owing to the fact I was 37 weeks pregnant but personal training sessions could be held in the comfort of your own home via Zoom. Then, after lockdown, it was because I realised a personal training session once a week meant I had a whole hour uninterrupted with no one shouting 'muuum' 173 times and the undivided attention of another grown-up. He asks me how I am, listens to what I say, and tells me I'm doing brilliantly every five minutes. What more can a mentally (over) loaded mama possibly want? So we've been going strong for 18 months and counting now. He says abs are made in the kitchen. After four babies I say they're not. Time will tell who's right.

"You always remember where you were and what you were doing when something momentous happens"

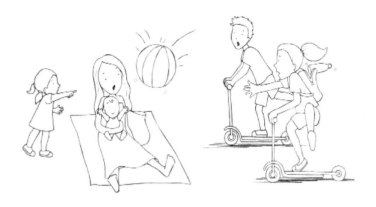

Chapter 11:

Mama Mia, Here We Go Again!

Confessions of an accidental mum of four: thin blue lines, a quaranteenie, and the support bubble I wouldn't pop for the world.

'**Y**ou've got your hands full' and 'don't you have a TV?' Those are among the uninvited remarks we seem to attract on an almost weekly basis since becoming a family of six. And what's more, strangers seem to find both comments side-splittingly funny. But because I hear them on an almost weekly basis I find them side-splittingly annoying. Along with being asked to repeat how many children we have because people either haven't heard correctly or can't quite believe it. Or both. So I smile politely and grit my teeth while shouting 'not four million, not four hundred, just *four!*' in my head.

Most people think we're mad for having four kids. And I don't blame them. I'm increasingly inclined to agree with them. I only know two other mamas of four, and they've both got four boys, so they *must* be mad. But the thing is we didn't plan it that way – it just happened. And it turns out there are all sorts of things we probably should have considered first, like how on earth to fit four car seats into the back of the car. And the pram. And the scooters. And the bikes. And how to cope when they're all crying at the same time. And what to do on the off-chance we find ourselves in the middle of a global pandemic.

So, after four babies - including an accidental lockdown one - here's what I wish I'd known about having a fourth baby:

1. Having (or wanting) lots of babies doesn't make you greedy.

And it doesn't make you selfish, either. Some people might think it does and that we should protect the planet by not having them, but I'm talking about something more primal than that.

After two consecutive miscarriages between Bluebell and Max – one at six weeks and one a 'missed' miscarriage at 11 weeks, when the baby's heart had stopped beating but there were no other signs anything was wrong – I wondered whether I was being greedy wanting another baby. I already had a healthy one, wasn't that enough? Was this God's way of telling me to be happy with what I already had?

When we then made it past the magic 12-week mark with Max I spent the entire pregnancy worried that something was going to go wrong as it had twice before. When he finally arrived and was safely in my arms (I pulled him to the surface of the birthing pool water myself - it mattered deeply that I should be his first human touch and that I should be the one to do this) I felt like a huge weight had been lifted off my shoulders. The feeling was so intense it was palpable. It was only then that I realised I'd spent the last nine months living under a cloud.

Then when I fell pregnant with Marigold (why *do* they call it that, as if you whoops-a-daisy slipped and fell) and later Violet I spent both pregnancies worried I was 'pushing my luck' and that I should have been grateful for what I already had, even though I am.

As a result, I dreaded all the scans, and my pregnancy scanxiety got worse with each baby. I was a nervous wreck by the time I had to have a 36-week presentation and position scan with Violet because they thought she was breech, made worse by the fact Misery Guts couldn't come with me because of Covid.

But having or wanting lots of babies *doesn't* make you greedy. It makes you a mama doing what your body was designed to do. And every baby is a blessing, whether it's your first, your fourth, or one that didn't quite make it and has wings somewhere in the sky.

2. It's easy to miss the tell-tale signs you're up the spout. Again.

You'd *think* after five pregnancies and three babies that I'd recognise the tell-tale signs we were expecting another baby, but no. In fact, the possibility of being pregnant with baby number four was so far from my mind I even googled 'reasons for nausea', thinking there might be something seriously wrong with me.

I *genuinely* couldn't work out why I was feeling so awful, and why I couldn't get rid of the metallic taste in my mouth no matter how many times I brushed my teeth. I couldn't work out why the bacon sandwich I ordered at soft play made me feel so sick. I couldn't work out why the smell of Misery Guts made me want to retch. And I couldn't work out why the sight of the washing mountain made me want to flip out and kill anyone who dared add anything to the top of it. *Especially* inside-out pants stuck inside inside-out trousers.

It wasn't until I was in Waitrose choosing a bottle of wine and wondering why I didn't fancy it that it finally dawned on me. I *never* don't fancy wine. So I left the wine in the wine aisle and went to the toiletries aisle where I picked up a pregnancy test instead of pinot. And you know how you always remember where you were and what you were doing when something momentous happens. Well, I was standing next to the dishwasher watching Misery Guts stack plates (wrongly) when I told him. And I'll never forget the look on his face. Or the number of times he repeated '*six!*' in a slightly crazed way when he realised it also meant we were going to become a family of six.

I'll also never forget that straight afterwards we had another inevitable you're-loading-the-dishwasher-wrong conversation like nothing momentous had happened. Why *can't* some people stack dishwashers properly? And why are they the same people who take the plastic stuff out and dump it on the draining board, instead of putting it away in the plastics cupboard where it belongs? Even though our plastics cupboard is overflowing it's still possible to open the door, throw another bit of plastic in, and shut it before everything inside comes tumbling out.

3. You think you've seen it all before – but you haven't.

Despite having been there, done it, and got the (sick stained) t-shirt three times before I thought I'd seen it all before and there was nothing more that could phase me when it came to having another baby. For example, it took me two babies to discover that the *real* reason for envelope sleeves on the shoulders of babygrows is so you can pull them down as well as up when a poonami strikes. Why don't they *tell* you that on the packet? Or have a diagram with arrows on at the very least? That would save *a lot* of poo-up-the-back-and-in-the-hair situations, a lot of wrestling them out of them, and a lot of bathing too.

I thought there was nothing more you could tell me that I didn't already know (or had found out the hard way) but I was wrong. Things have progressed. A lot. Like gold poppers at the centre of babygrows so you know which one is the middle and you can start there first. Thus avoiding poppering the whole thing up only to discover you missed one and having to undo it all and repopper again. Whoever came up with that idea is quite frankly a *genius*.

I also thought there was nothing you could tell me that I didn't already know (or had found out the hard way) about being pregnant. But it turns out it's easy to *completely* forget what it's like being pregnant until you are again. Apart from feeling sick, that unexplained metallic taste in the mouth, aversion to smells including your other half, and mummy mood swings, I'd also forgotten what it's like to feel all first trimesterish, even when you're not in the first trimester anymore. And the eye-watering heartburn even though you've eaten and done nothing to warrant it. And the fact that you're actually going to have (another) baby at the end of it.

Somewhere between baby number one and baby number four I also became what's known as a geriatric mum. Phrases like 'advanced maternal age' started (rather alarmingly) appearing on my maternity notes when I wasn't even 40, although admittedly I was in my fortieth year by the time I had Violet. While I'm the first to admit that motherhood has aged me in ways I could never have imagined, I do think the word geriatric is going a bit far.

4. Counting becomes second nature.

I do it every time we leave the house or get into the car because I'm terrified of 'forgetting' one of them.

Misery Guts reckons it's only a matter of time, and I *totally* get how David Cameron left one of his in the pub. I even have anxiety dreams about it and wake up counting children we don't even have.

It's not just me doing the counting either. When we go out in public I can see people mentally counting us. Every. Single. Time. Sometimes they even do a re-count, starting with the pushchair and then the older ones on their bikes and scooters. Then seeing them mentally counting us makes me panic and count us all again, just to be certain we haven't left someone somewhere. We haven't – yet (unless you include accidentally leaving Violet in the car once but it was seconds not minutes and we were yards not metres away so I don't think that counts) - but like Misery Guts says, it's probably only a matter of time.

5. There's no such thing as a family ticket.

As a family of five we didn't fit into the 'two adults, two kids' family ticket criteria anyway, but now we're a family of six it appears we've broken the mould. I routinely nearly choke on my tea (or wine depending on what time of day it is) when I discover how much family days out are going to cost once you've taken into account all the various tickets required. And as if paying through the nose for everything isn't bad enough, it makes the disappointment and dismay worse if the day out in question turns out not to be worth the cash. Which happens quite a lot.

Being a family of six was also a bit of a problem when it came to the rule of six during the pandemic. The problem with the rule of six when you already *are* six was that it didn't make a blind bit of difference. We still couldn't meet up with family and friends from another household indoors or outdoors and introduce our quaranteenie to the world.

What I didn't (and still don't) understand is how Violet could possibly be classed as one of the six. As a newborn she couldn't go anywhere on her own, interact with anyone on her own or do anything independently. She was essentially an extension of me. (Interestingly, the rule of six was different in Scotland and Wales and kids weren't included).

I also didn't (and still don't) understand how the kids could go to school and nursery and swimming and gymnastics and Brownies as usual but we couldn't see both grandparents from the same household at the same time. It was absurd. And don't even get me started on the fact that hunting and grouse shooting were also exempt from the rule of six because it was classed as a 'sports gathering'. There is no question that being out and about with four kids running in opposite directions and two parents and two grandparents trying to catch them could also be classed as a sports gathering.

6. Everything has to be *exactly* the same.

Even Violet can clock within seconds whether she's been given a plate of food or a drink that isn't *exactly* the same as her brother and sisters. Where *does* that outrage come from?

There's absolutely no point getting each of them a different flavour ice cream or a different colour balloon – everything has to be the same or it's 'not fair' and all hell breaks loose. What's more, any slight variation in colour, size, or style will be noted and held against you for the rest of your life, to the point you wish you'd never bothered in the first place.

7. There's a thin blue line between harmony and total chaos.

Or four thin blue lines. And you pick your battles. Like letting your fournado go on a muddy country walk in pink glittery sandals even though you know they'll have to go in the bin afterwards. Because it's just not worth the showdown if you don't. And you even help her search for them when she discovers they're missing, even though you know full well you've thrown them away and they're long gone at the bottom of a bin somewhere. Because it's just easier that way.

It's also easier to let her go to nursery dressed as Belle from Beauty and the Beast even though the costume is made from 100% polyester and it's the hottest day of the year so far. And it's easier to let her wear her Christmas jumper every day of the year *except* Christmas jumper day because for some reason no one can fathom she suddenly refuses to wear it on Christmas jumper day even though it's for charity. And it's easier to only bath her once a week because washing her hair is such a nightmare. I think third child syndrome is the correct name for it.

8. You have to accept that at some point you're going to have to choose between them.

It's inevitable. I don't mean picking a favourite child, I mean deciding whose need is the greatest. For example, what to do when they're all crying at the same time. When I was a mum of two I thought two kids crying at the same time was bad but try three – or all four. It's got to be seen – and heard – to be believed.

Who do you go to first? The youngest? The loudest? The one with blood? The one with the poo in places there shouldn't be poo? And what's worse – blood or poo? And what about sick? Is sick better or worse than blood or poo, or is it about the same? The struggle is real. All these questions then beg a really serious question. Like who you would save first. And I don't have an answer for that.

And the thing is you're damned if you do and you're damned if you don't anyway because one person can't deal with four little people all at the same time. Two people can't either. The odds are well and truly stacked against you.

Things also seem to happen that didn't happen when you weren't outnumbered and had (slightly) more control. Like the baby eating crusts of toast they've extracted from the bin which you later discover was next to a dirty nappy you hadn't put in a sack because you were too busy being outnumbered. And number two telling number three to lick his verruca and she does it, even though she doesn't do anything else anyone tells her. Ever. You also find yourself getting quite shouty. Because there's only so many times you can say 'put your shoes on' and 'brush your teeth' without flipping out.

9. You'll develop a love-hate relationship with kids TV.

When you first start watching kids' TV after a gap since your own childhood it's a bit like entering a whole new universe. Not only is kids TV on *all* the time on multiple channels at the touch of a button - as opposed to after lunch and for a couple of hours after school with a test card in between - which I found quite frankly mind-blowing, it's a very weird, psychedelic universe involving things like pontipines, ninky nonks, and twirlywoos. As we've already established in the myth of having it all and confessions of a mama doing too many things and none of them well it's best not to overthink these things, otherwise you can find yourself having some very dark thoughts, like CBeebies dark thoughts, which is an actual hashtag on Twitter.

Yet it's hard *not* to think about it when they show some of the programmes twice a day and you've had to endure them with four different kids. Like how the family set up in Peppa Pig can *possibly* be setting a good example when Daddy Pig is constantly referred to as 'silly daddy' and is such a nincompoop. He's basically a useless, bumbling DIY disaster who can't read a map, and much of what he does goes wrong, which is then put right by the all-knowing and competent Mummy Pig. What is this teaching the next generation?

And why *is* Topsy and Tim's mum so happy and twintastically smug and perfect? Misery Guts reckons she's up to no good with DIY Derek because when you actually watch it she's always 'popping out' and there are rather a lot of unexplained absences.

The so-called classic children's stories, most of which have now made it on to screen too, aren't much better either. Like Sophie's mum in the Tiger Who Came To Tea. The look on her face when she realises there's nothing for daddy's tea because the tiger ate it all makes me want to slap her. Perish the thought of daddy actually making his own dinner.

But 10 years and four babies later I find myself getting quite nostalgic when programmes that Bluebell watched when she was a baby come on and entertain Violet in the same way they did her big sister. I used to hate Mr Tumble, but now I could hug him. Ditto Daddy Pig. I still can't work out why Topsy and Tim's mum is so twintastically happy though. Or whether she really *is* having it off with DIY Derek.

10. You know when you're done mumming – and when you're not.

They say never say never. And while I've already admitted in confessions from the lady with the boobs that I wouldn't rule out a bit of help in the decolletage department after breastfeeding four babies, I can categorically say we will never have another baby.

If there's one question we've been asked the most since becoming a family of six it's whether we'll be having any more, and I have a one-word answer: no! I love them to the moon and back and my heart is bursting, but our family is *very* definitely complete.

Because you know when you're 'done' doing something. After Marigold was born I definitely didn't feel like I was done having babies yet. I loved the idea of a fourth baby and knew I had it in me to do it all again, but Misery Guts made no secret of the fact he didn't. So I resigned myself to the fact that only winning the lottery might persuade him otherwise, and that we were stopping at three.

In hindsight, I can see that the reason I mourned giving up breastfeeding Marigold so much and had my breast milk turned into jewellery and even went to a boob printing workshop was because I thought I'd never get the chance to do it all again.

I can also see that the fact I'm *not* mourning the idea of giving up breastfeeding Violet and that folding and putting away her baby clothes doesn't make me want to cry means I'm definitely done mumming this time.

That said, knowing I'm done mumming didn't stop me shoehorning Violet into her pram at six months old, two months after she outgrew it. Because I know I'll never push a baby of my own in a pram again. And things happen when you push a pram, things that don't happen when you push a pushchair or you're chasing behind a toddler on a scooter.

Aside from the fact that pushing a pram makes you feel like a *proper* grown-up, people stand aside to let you pass. Which is super helpful if you're always late like me. You can also fit everything but the kitchen sink in it. Which is super helpful if they've got 25 per cent off six bottles of wine at the supermarket.

Knowing when you're done mumming and not having any more babies is a bittersweet decision in many ways, but for us I know it's the right one. They're the support bubble I wouldn't pop for the world. Even if the wheels do fall off now and again.

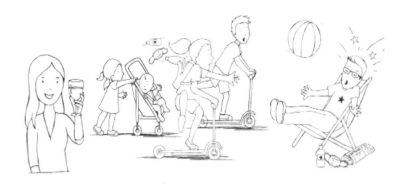

Chapter 12:

Our roadmap to freedom
(with a few burst bubbles along the way)

Confessions of a corona mummy: learning to go with the (lateral) flow, false positives, and surviving a global pandemic.

How do pandemics end? That's what Max (six) asked me one rainy day in lockdown. It's a jolly good question – and yet another one I didn't have the answer to. (I asked Alexa and she didn't know, either). Apparently, pandemics fade and peter out, and at the time of writing I *think* we've managed to survive one.

There's absolutely no doubt accidentally having a fourth baby in the middle of a global pandemic was crap, and I wouldn't recommend it. Not the fourth baby - like the others, she's a little piece of me I didn't know was missing - I mean the pandemic. Other than high days and holidays, I never *dreamed* we'd all be at home at the same time for months on end without anyone being able to go anywhere, see anyone, or do anything. The idea of the world shutting down was inconceivable, and at eight months pregnant and with three kids suddenly at home, I thought it was the end of the world.

Of course, it wasn't the end of the world. There were even some positives to lockdown too. Like there being no need to pull the drawbridge up in order to secure the much-feted fourth trimester with Violet. The drawbridge was already up. There was also no need to make up excuses because you weren't up to visitors yet – or because you simply didn't want to see them. There was no one to judge if I was walking around in maternity leggings with holes in and baby sick on my shoulder, and there wasn't even any need to do up my nursing bra clips.

So, after four babies - including an accidental lockdown one - here's what I wish I'd known about parenting in a pandemic:

1. If you can survive pandemic parenting you can survive anything.

And one day we will look back and laugh. Even about homeschooling. Although probably not about improper fractions. Or armpit fudge. Or back to school shopping with a licky five-year-old. Because if you can survive pandemic parenting, you can survive anything. And we all deserve a medal, whether we rode out the storm in a yacht, in a canoe, or by (almost) drowning.

For us lockdown was a crazy and completely unsustainable mix of home learning grids, nappy changing, fronted adverbials, improper fractions, 'teaching' from the sofa while breastfeeding, shouting at the printer, and trying to suppress the inner rage that started building well before nine o'clock every weekday morning. Some days just keeping everyone alive without killing each other was an achievement. And we won't take supermarket home delivery slots for granted again, either.

Yet post-pandemic, having done all that and (just about) survived, I can confidently say I've got this, even though I still don't know what 'it' actually is, and probably never will. And that's ok.

2. You have to learn to go with the (lateral) flow.

Because a global pandemic is out of your control. Which is a bit of a problem if you like to be *in* control. I learnt this at the very start of the first lockdown when I realised I'd be giving birth in the middle of a global pandemic and no one really knew what was going on, least of all my midwife. And it was a good lesson given what was to come.

When I think back to the early days of the first lockdown the phrase 'the blind leading the blind' springs to mind. The truth is we were all winging it – the Government, teachers, employers, parents. All you can do is your best and if sometimes that isn't good enough (and it really wasn't) then so be it. You had to learn to go with the (lateral) flow.

Thankfully it was still possible to cheer yourself up by buying things on the internet. One of the first things I did when the schools and nurseries closed and my maternity leave was hijacked and the true awfulness of what was about to happen dawned on me was buy the pram I'd *always* wanted but we could never afford. We still couldn't afford it, but I reasoned the maternity leave tea and cake I wouldn't be buying in coffee shops and the days out we wouldn't be having could pay for it. And because lockdown went on for as long as it did, it did.

3. Burst bubbles are inevitable.

Especially when you've got a licky five-year-old with absolutely no concept of a link between his tongue, germs, and a global pandemic on your hands. In fact, I'm surprised the bubbles in our house didn't burst more often than they did.

I think we got off lightly compared to some areas where bubbles were bursting all over town and families were forced to self-isolate, and no sooner was one period of self-isolation over than you were forced to start another.

A burst bubble did prompt me to spend our child benefit on a private Covid test kit though. It all started with The Call, the one I knew we'd get at some point. The kids had been back at school and nursery for just one week after Lockdown 1 when nursery called to say Marigold had started coughing and could we come and collect her. Despite having what we were 99.9% certain was a common cold, she wasn't allowed to return to nursery until she had tested negative for coronavirus. Which was easier said than done.

Unless we were able to travel 735 miles away to John

O'Groats there were no tests available in our area (the NHS website *insisted* John O'Groats was just 4.1 miles away, and no matter how many times I told them it wasn't the computer said no). And no-one seemed to know when – or even if – more tests would be delivered. And as we all now know a coronavirus test must be carried out within five days of a person displaying symptoms, otherwise it is assumed the person in question is positive and their entire household must quarantine for 10 days.

The thought of all six of us living in a two-bedroom flat with no garden for 10 days while continuing to pay for childcare we weren't using, after school clubs the kids couldn't go to, and try to work at the same time was more than I could bear, so I spent £149 great British pounds – more than half of our monthly child benefit – on a private Covid test kit instead.

When it arrived I felt like I had won one of Willy Wonka's golden tickets. As predicted the cough was a common cold and Marigold was back to nursery the next day.

Until the next bubble burst, that is.

4. Don't panic about false positives.

Like messages from nursery starting with the line 'We've had a positive case of...' prompting you to panic and click on it only to discover they're talking about chickenpox or whooping cough, not coronavirus.

Pre-Covid a case of chickenpox or whooping cough would have sparked widespread panic, especially among working parents. The WhatsApp group and breakout WhatsApp groups would have gone into meltdown with messages from parents whose first names you can't quite remember because you stupidly saved their number as 'Darcy's mum', as though they don't have their own independent existence, and now it's too late to ask them what their name is. All while you try to sort out alternative childcare and debate whether it's simply best to throw a chickenpox party and get it all over and done with.

But post-Covid chickenpox or whooping cough is the least of our worries. Once the worst possible scenario, either option is now the best. I also discovered it's also a good idea to (temporarily) unmute the class WhatsApp groups – and the breakout ones – so you can be among the first to discover when a bubble has burst and you have to go and pick them up, instead of the last. And when I say last I mean five hours later last. Because discovering that during those five hours they've been sat in an office on their own waiting for you to pick them up can make you feel like a *really* terrible mum.

5. Finding our new normal after lockdown was bittersweet.

They say you never remember the last time you change a nappy or the last time you wipe down a highchair, but I remember exactly the last time I climbed back into bed with a cup of tea and lay Violet on my chest after getting Bluebell, Max, and Marigold off to school and nursery in the morning. It was Friday, December 18th, 2020, the day term time ended and school and nursery broke up for Christmas.

Little did I know then that it would be almost three months until I had the chance to climb back into bed with a cup of tea and lay Violet on my chest again, but that when that time came I wouldn't be able to because she'd grown too big. Thanks to Lockdown 3 Bluebell and Max didn't go back to school until March 2021, and during that time Violet not only learnt to roll over but sit up but crawl too. And she didn't even fit on my chest anymore.

I should have been celebrating these milestones – and I did - but I can't help but also mourn all the time we didn't have together when she was tiny. Little moments like snuggling in bed before she was mobile when instead I was grappling with 'new maths' and trying to get my head around the bus stop method. Which makes finding a new normal after Lockdown 3 really bittersweet.

6. Lockdown wasn't all bad.

It was pretty bad, but it wasn't *all* bad. There are actually some things I'm going to miss about lockdown. Which is a sentence I never thought I'd write. Like kitchen discos, rainbows, and Gary Barlow's Crooner Sessions. (I won't miss banana bread or garden igloos though).

A lockdown silver lining had to be the slower pace of life and not having to wake up with an alarm, get everyone out of the door by a certain time, and constantly check the time to see where we were supposed to be next. It's fair to say we're not morning people.

I also found myself questioning how much of our 'old life' I actually wanted to go back to because for the first time in years lockdown forced us to take our foot off the pedal and slow down, something that simply wouldn't have happened otherwise. It also made me realise just how crazy bonkers our pre-coronavirus lives actually were what with work, school, nursery, and after-school clubs.

Lockdown highlights in our house included dancing to Queen with wooden spoons for microphones in the kitchen with Bluebell and Marigold; painting rainbows on pebbles from the beach with Max; and of course the arrival of our own little rainbow Violet Hope. I don't know about you, but I'll always associate rainbows with the year the world paused.

7. Lockdown taught me *a lot* about my family.

Like the fact that kids thrive on routine, and all hell breaks loose through lack of it. And that Max has an unhealthy fascination with bums, especially his own. And that I cannot fathom how four children brought up in exactly the same way under exactly the same roof can be so different.

At first, I balked at the homemade schedules being shared on the class WhatsApp groups and social media – especially the laminated ones - but after a few weeks I started to get it. I needed laminated schedules in my life too. Or even better, someone to tell me what to do with them.

It was around then that we hit on the idea of introducing marbles as a reward for good behaviour. Because otherwise I was in danger of losing my marbles. So I bought a bag of marbles on the internet and every time the kids did as they were told they earned a marble. We put them in a glass jar and when the jar was full they got a prize (you guessed it – more stuff from the internet). It worked a treat until I discovered they'd been stealing marbles from each other's jars and putting them in their own. So I stole them all, put them in my own jar, bought myself my own prize on the internet and that was the end of that.

Lockdown also taught me that and clarinets and recorders should be left at school. They *shouldn't* be practiced in two-bedroom flats. Especially when the player is nine and only knows how to 'play' one song.

8. Seesawing my way through a pandemic has left me with a post-traumatic stress-style twitch.

A little muscle in the left-hand corner of my left eye starts twitching at the mere mention of the word Seesaw. And when Seesaw notifications appear on my phone, my heart starts racing. Presumably I'll get over it as time goes on and the awfulness of homeschooling fades, but if I ever see another Seesaw printout again it will be too soon.

The first thing I did when the kids went back to school after Lockdown 3 was cleanse and reclaim my home office. It took three bin bags, most of which contained the dreaded Seesaw printouts. There were a few things I couldn't bear to part with though, including the scale model of an Egyptian pyramid (it had a sliding door on it and everything). Unfortunately I can't claim any credit for it – it miraculously appeared after my mum and dad stepped in to help.

Our homeschooling performance was summed up rather succinctly in Max's end of year school report, which stated 'family circumstances made remote learning very difficult so we are unable to grade engagement'. By which they meant accidentally having a fourth baby in the middle of a global pandemic meant I was doing too many things and none of them well. I felt like *I* was the one being assessed, not Max. And that made the little muscle in the left-hand corner of my left eye twitch even more.

I was so cross that our homeschooling performance – or lack of it - had been assessed in the same way lessons at school were assessed that I started an irate email in response once the kids were in bed. Fuelled by pinot, I angrily bashed out why it wasn't fair that homeschooling was included in the school reports when home circumstances vary so wildly. At school children are given the same opportunities and are therefore assessed from a level playing field. How can the homeschooling performance of an only child with a stay-at-home mum or dad *possibly* be compared to a child with one or more siblings whose parents both work? Or a single parent who works? Or a mum of four with an accidental lockdown baby who's supposed to be on maternity leave?

I already know I did a bad job. But it was the best I could do with two totally different remote learning timetables, a three-year-old and a newborn while recovering from giving birth and dealing with the subsequent and inevitable sleep deprivation. Now I've got a school report on headed paper to prove it. Of course the email is still saved as a draft in my inbox, because I ran out of steam (and pinot), got distracted, and then it seemed like too much time had passed to send it. The little muscle in the left-hand corner of my left eye still twitches when I think about it though.

9. You have to divide and conquer.

Especially when it comes to getting around the rule of six when you already *are* six. Once lockdown restrictions started to ease most outings involved cutting ourselves in half, with Misery Guts meeting up with friends and family and going somewhere and doing something with two kids, and me meeting up with friends and family and going somewhere and doing something with the other two. And after being cooped up inside together for the best part of a year the break from each other was a bit of a relief.

Dividing and conquering is probably the best way forward for us as an outnumbered family of six now anyway, because the dynamic changes when you've only got one or two kids to keep in check instead of three – or four. And dividing and conquering is *definitely* the best way forward when it comes to back-to-school shopping, pandemic or no pandemic. From now on I will only undertake back-to-school shopping with one child at a time. Even if that means it takes the best part of a week to get the job done.

10. The baby years are fleeting – and even more fleeting in a pandemic.

They say the first twelve months go by in the blink of an eye, and they really do. But it turns out they go by even faster in a pandemic. We might have been locked down (or up, depending on which way you look at it) together for the best part of Violet's first year but the days and weeks went by in a blink of homeschooling, procrastibaking, trying to book online Big Shops, hanging out of the living room window banging pots and pans for the NHS, watching five o'clock Downing Street briefings and trying not to catch Covid.

It was only a matter of time until one of us did, ironically a full 18 months later as I proofread these final pages. Which given the licky five-year-old situation and the fact the kids will *still* quite happily chase a dough ball across a restaurant floor is nothing short of a miracle.

If I could turn the clock back and do it all again with each of my babies I would, but I'd do it all again with Violet especially as we were robbed of so much time together and you just can't have that time back again. It's true what they say: the days are long but the years are short. They also say you lose yourself in motherhood – and to some extent that's true. But the truth is I also found myself. Even in the middle of a global pandemic.

The End.

(Except it isn't the end. It's only just the beginning...)

Thank yous

If you'd asked me when I was little what I wanted to be when I grew up I would have said an author. I used to sit in front of my grandpa's electric typewriter in my grandparents' summer house in East Sussex dreaming about the amazing story I was going to write, even though I didn't know what it was going to be about yet. If I think hard enough I can still smell that typewriter. And the summer house.

I spent my twenties and most of my thirties still dreaming about the amazing story I was going to write, even though I didn't know what it was going to be about yet. But somehow life - and little people - got in the way, and it remained a dream that I'd think about every now and again when I had a spare moment. Which wasn't very often. Then one day in lockdown when the whole world paused it dawned on me. The blog I'd started as a first time mum, when I had lots to say and no-one to say it to and had faithfully updated every week for the last seven years, *was* a book. It was the book I didn't know I'd written. Accidentally having a fourth baby in the middle of a global pandemic was the hook I needed to transform the virtual pages of Confessions of a Crummy Mummy into the pages of a real book. The amazing story I was going to write wasn't going to be a figment of my imagination. It was going to be real life. Because when it comes to parenting – *especially* pandemic parenting – you simply couldn't make it up.

So I looked back at everything I'd written over the last seven years and set about turning Confessions of a Crummy Mummy the blog into Confessions of a Crummy Mummy the book with a beginning, a middle and an end. I got up early and stayed up late when everyone else was asleep, I wrote one-handed on my phone with my non-dominant hand while breastfeeding Violet, and I added bits in and took bits out while cooking the tea and trying to get my head around improper fractions. Slowly but surely, amid the chaos of lockdown, hijacked maternity leave, homeschooling, and trying to find the right Zoom codes, the amazing story I was going to write started to take shape and Confessions of a Crummy Mummy – The Baby Years was born. (Of course, it's up to you to decide whether it really *is* amazing or not!)

I always imagined dedicating my amazing story to my grandpa for being the first person to encourage me to write at his electric typewriter in the summer house in East Sussex. But he'd turn in his grave if he knew I'd written about fanny farts and foo-foos and (almost) giving a condom to a Beaver. I don't think he'd think it's an amazing story, either. He'd think I was unashamedly oversharing things best kept to oneself, and he'd be absolutely right. He was always right.

But the thing is it isn't written for him. It's written for you, and me, and all the mamas feeling like they're doing too many things and none of them well. We're all in it together and I wanted this book to be a celebration of that. That and perfectly imperfect parenting. Whether you've been with me since the beginning or you're new (hello!) thank you – this book wouldn't have been possible without you and your follows, likes, comments, hearts, and shares.

So instead of my grandpa it seemed fitting to dedicate my amazing story to those I've got to thank for the fanny farts and foo-foo tales and (almost) giving a condom to a Beaver. It's true what I said at the very beginning – my amazing story wouldn't have been possible without Bluebell, Maxi, Marigold, Violet, and of course Misery Guts. You are all a piece of me that I didn't know was missing and this is the story of us. It's *our* amazing story. (While we're on the subject of Misery Guts, he might be grumpy and get in a mood when I ask him to take zillions of pictures so I can pick 'the one' to share with you lovely lot but he's also my weathervane, partner in alphabites crime and there's no-one else I'd rather do it all with. Except maybe

Robbie Williams, but don't tell him. Don't tell Misery Guts, either).

Thanks must also go to my wonderful team of beta readers – you know who you are! Thank you for your time, honesty, thoughts, suggestions, and verdicts, which you'll find at the front of this book. I felt physically sick when I first sent you the manuscript, waited with bated breath while you read it and cried (in a good way!) when you gave me your feedback.

Thanks also to my agent Susan Mears, her wonderful assistant Hayley Finch, and my publisher Chris Day. Firstly for your enthusiasm about my amazing story idea, then for believing I had it in me to actually write it, and then for holding my hand throughout the whole process. And to the fabulously talented Helen Braid for her wonderful illustrations and helping to make my amazing story look like a real book with real pictures in a way that only you could – thank you! To say the last year has been a learning curve is an understatement.

It's also a dream come true, and if I could go back to seven-year-old me in my grandpa's summer house in East Sussex I'd tell her to never stop dreaming about the amazing story she was going to write, even though she doesn't know what it's going to be about yet. Because 34 years later here it is in your hands –

the amazing story I was going to write. (Or *I* think it's amazing anyway, given the circumstances and being outnumbered and always feeling like I'm doing too many things and none of them well). And now I'm not only a wife, mother, freelance journalist, and blogger, but finally an author too.

If you liked my amazing story (or even if you didn't – I don't mind!) please feel free to pop by and say hello – you can find me unashamedly oversharing life as an accidental mum of four at www.crummymummy.co.uk, on Instagram and Facebook (@confessionsofacrummymummy) and on Twitter (@mrsnataliebrown).

Printed in Great Britain
by Amazon